A Guide
Health Care Providers

The Chiari Book:
A Guide for Patients, Families, and Health Care Providers

THE CHIARI I MALFORMATION AND SYRINGOMYELIA

John J. Oro, Diane Mueller

2007

Copyright © 2007 John J. Oro, Diane Mueller
All rights reserved.
ISBN: 1-4196-4642-7
ISBN-13: 978-1419646423
Library of Congress Control Number: 2006907059

The Chiari Book:
A Guide for Patients, Families, and Health Care Providers

CONTENTS

1.	Introduction	1
2.	A brief review of Neuroanatomy	5
3.	The Chiari Malformations	11
4.	Syringomyelia	21
5.	Symptoms of Chiari I Malformation	27
6.	Other Illnesses That Can Mimic Chiari I Malformation	33
7.	The Diagnosis of Chiari I Malformation and Syringomyelia	39
8.	Treatment Options for Chiari I Malformation and Syringomyelia	49
9.	Special Considerations in Chiari (children and adolescents, pregnancy, elderly)	57
10.	Summary	63

APPENDICES:

Chiari and Syringomyelia Articles	65
Glossary	89
Internet Resources	95

Acknowledgements

We are grateful to our colleagues at the University of Missouri Health Sciences Center and Columbia Regional Hospital for their collaboration in the care of patients with Chiari and syringomyelia. We also thank the colleagues at The Medical Center of Aurora and staff at the Chiari Care Center that are helping expand the services delivered to patients suffering from these disorders. We offer special thanks to Suzanne Oro, for the proof reading and editing of the manuscript, as well as coordinating its publication.

"This book is dedicated to all of those who suffer from Chiari Malformation and syringomyelia, their families, and caregivers."

CHAPTER 1

INTRODUCTION

The Chiari (pronounced kee are ee) Type I malformation (CMI) is an uncommon, congenital, neuroskeletal deformity that can cause a great variety of neurological symptoms. A quick look at structure of the skull and brain will help better understand the disorder. The brain exists in a hollow space surrounded by bone. The brainstem and cerebellum normally sit in a funnel-like cavity just above the spinal cord (Figure 1).

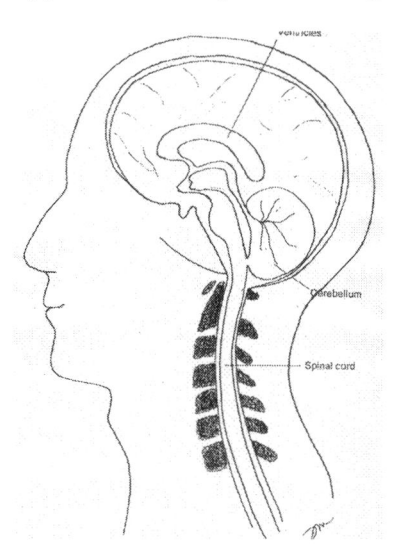

Figure 1: Normal brainstem anatomy, showing the cerebellum in a normal position.

The Chiari I malformation is believed to occur when the back compartment of the skull, called the *posterior fossa,* is not formed properly. The cerebellar tonsils are structures at the bottom of the cerebellum (Figure 2). Instead of sitting in their proper space, the tonsils are displaced downward into the funnel, thus causing pressure on the lower part of the brain and upper cervical spinal cord. The flow of *cerebrospinal fluid* (CSF) through this area is blocked because the brain tissue is stuffed into this funnel. Sometimes the tonsils appear shrunken (*atrophic*) and may stick to the spinal cord. This downward displacement of the cerebellar tonsils causing crowding is called the Chiari I malformation.

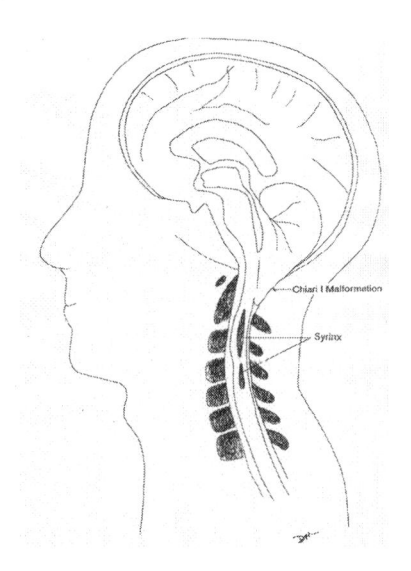

Figure 2: Abnormal brainstem anatomy, showing the cerebellar tonsils herniated beyond the foramen magnum and crowding the CSF space. Image also shows syrinx cavities in the cervical spinal cord.

The exact cause of the Chiari I malformation is not known. The malformation is likely to occur during the early embryonic development of the brainstem and spinal cord. An abnormally small posterior fossa results in the tonsils, and sometimes the brainstem, being forced downward. The defect can occur in infants, children and adolescents. However, more commonly, it causes problems in adults. For reasons that are not known, the Chiari I malformation occurs more often in women than men.

Some people with Chiari I malformation also have a syrinx (se-ri-nx), or syringomyelia, a cavity (or pocket) within the spinal cord containing CSF. Syringomyelia is not always associated with Chiari I malformation, and may occur in spinal cord trauma, infections, tumors, or for unknown reasons. It is not known why syringomyelia develops, but in persons with the Chiari I malformation it is related to obstruction of spinal fluid flow caused by the crowding at the opening at the base of the skull. This blockage results in an abnormal spinal fluid flow leading to spinal fluid collecting inside the spinal cord. These structural changes, the Chiari I malformation with or without syringomyelia, can affect many kinds of nerves and brain tissues resulting in a wide variety of neurological symptoms. These will be detailed in chapter 5.

CHAPTER 2

A BRIEF REVIEW OF NEUROANATOMY

The brain is enclosed and protected by a rounded skull made of bone. The inside of the skull is partly separated into two compartments, a large upper compartment which includes the two upper halves of the brain known as *cerebral hemispheres* and a smaller (and lower) compartment at the back of the head known as the *posterior fossa*. The lower part includes the *brain stem* and *cerebellum*. The brain stem continues through an opening at the bottom of the skull, called the *foramen magnum*, where it connects to the *spinal cord*.

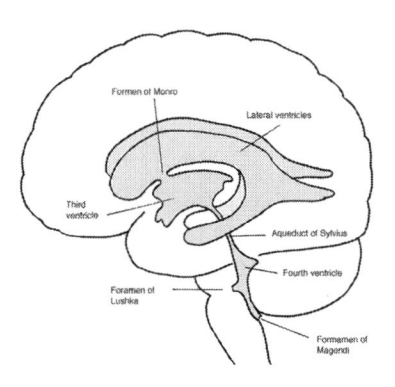

Figure 1: Side view of the brain showing the cerebral ventricles.

There are four spaces (or pockets) filled with spinal fluid within the brain called *ventricles* (Figure 1). Two large C-shaped ventricles, the *lateral ventricles*, are located within the cerebral hemispheres and drain into the *third ventricle*. From the third ventricle spinal fluid flows through a small tunnel (the *aqueduct of Sylvius*) into the *fourth ventricle* located between the brain stem and cerebellum. Spinal fluid then flows from the fourth ventricle through three openings: two openings at the side of the fourth ventricle (the *foramina of Lushka*), and one at the bottom of the fourth ventricle (the *foramen of Magendie*). Through these three foramina (openings) spinal fluid flows to the surface of the brain and down the spinal canal.

Spinal fluid is created by a tuft or clump of vascular tissue called the *choroid plexus,* which is present within each ventricle. With every heartbeat, blood passing in the choroid plexus is filtered to create a clear colorless fluid that looks like water and is called *cerebral spinal fluid,* or *CSF*. Once spinal fluid flows down through the ventricles and around the brain and spinal cord, it is taken back up through large veins, most located at the top of the brain. Here it becomes part of the blood that drains through the jugular veins and goes to the heart. Each time the heart beats a small amount of spinal fluid is created inside the ventricles at the same time a small amount of spinal fluid is taken up by the veins, keeping the system in balance.

The Spinal Fluid Cisterns

The spinal fluid cushions the brain and spinal cord from injury. It flows through different pockets on the surfaces of the brain called *cisterns*. An important cistern, the *cisterna magna,* is located at the bottom of the skull (Figure 2). The word *magna*, meaning great or large in Latin, reminds us that the cisterna magna is the largest of the cisterns. This cistern is important because most of the spinal fluid flowing from the ventricles drains into it on its way to the spinal canal and the surface of the brain. Crowding of the cisterna magna, such as in the Chiari I malformation, can block the normal flow of spinal fluid.

Structures in the Posterior Fossa and Upper Spinal Canal

The posterior fossa contains three important neurological structures: the brain stem, cranial nerves, and cerebellum. The *brain stem* contains the nerve centers controlling eye movements, feeling and movement of the face, hearing, swallowing, shrugging the shoulders, and movement of the tongue. From these centers (nuclei) run the *cranial nerves* that travel through small holes at the bottom of the skull to and from their area of activity. The brainstem also contains nerve centers controlling heart and breathing functions.

The *cerebellum* is attached to the back of the brainstem and regulates coordination and the ability to move smoothly. Disorders of the cerebellum include an unsteady walk, coordination problems, and difficulty with fine motor tasks such as buttoning a shirt. Like the cerebrum, the cerebellum is divided into two hemispheres. As is noted in Figure 2, the bottom portions of the cerebellar hemisphere are the *cerebellar tonsils* (different from the tonsils located in the throat).

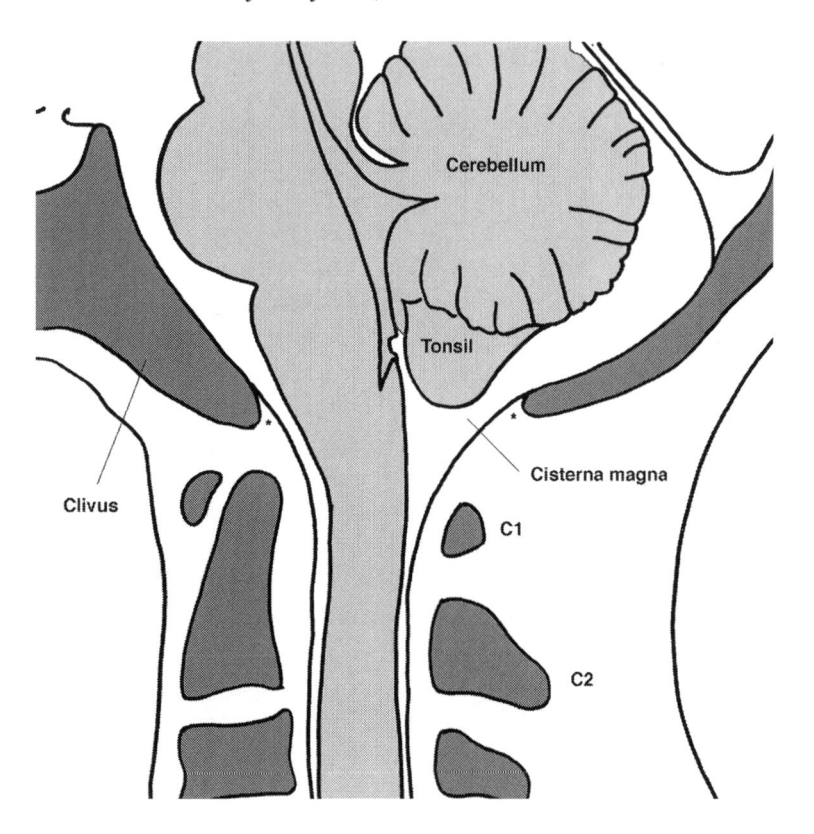

Figure 2: Side view of a normal posterior fossa. The triangular shaped bone in front of the brain stem is called the *clivus*. The skull bone at the back of the cerebellum is called the *supraocciput*. The *foramen magnum* is the opening between the tip of the clivus bone and the tip of the supraocciput bone (small dots). The *cisterna magna* is behind and below the tonsils of the cerebellum. (Adapted from Barrow Neurological Institute Quarterly)

The brain stem joins the spinal cord at the level of the foramen magnum. Inside the spinal cord run nerve fibers controlling movement of the arms, trunk, legs and bowel and bladder function. The spinal cord lies within the spinal canal, which is surrounded by the bony vertebrae. The upper most vertebrae is called cervical one, (or C1) and the second is cervical two (C2). There are a total of seven cervical vertebrae in the neck.

CHAPTER 3

THE CHIARI MALFORMATIONS

In 1891, Dr Hans Chiari, a German pathologist, described a series of defects or malformations at the base of the brain, and described them as "hindbrain herniation". The malformations were found on autopsy examination, and now bear his name- the Chiari malformations. Approximately 4 years later, Dr Arnold also studied the hindbrain herniations, and, for many years the malformations were known as the Arnold-Chiari malformations. However, it is now understood that Dr Arnold did not significantly add to the original description of the disorder and they are now simply referred to as the Chiari malformations.

The Chiari malformations are a complex, neuroskeletal deformities presumed to be present at birth. There are three types of Chiari malformations.

The **Chiari type I malformation (CMI)** is the most common type of Chiari malformation. The Chiari malformation is believed to occur when the posterior fossa is formed improperly during fetal development, and the space is too small to hold all the contents. Type I malformation has previously been defined as herniation of the cerebellar tonsils 3mm-5mm or more below the level of the foramen magnum, although we now know that some patients with less herniation or descent may still have symptoms. The amount of herniation is measured by an imaginary line drawn across the foramen magnum (Line

A in Figure 1). Crowding of the contents of the posterior fossa results in downward displacement of the cerebellar tonsils, causing obstruction of cerebrospinal fluid (CSF) flow. The cerebellar tonsils normally end a few millimeters above the foramen magnum on MRI. In the Chiari I malformation, the tonsils hang downward and may appear pointed or peg-like due to pressure on the tissue. This downward displacement and the crowding it causes is defined as the Chiari I malformation.

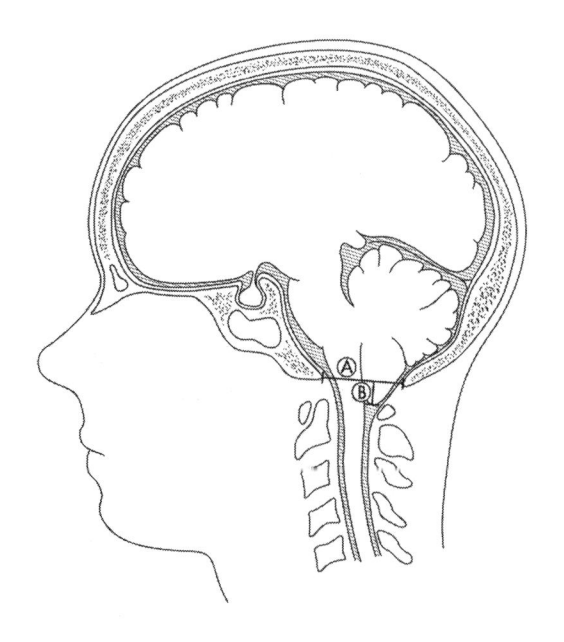

Figure 1: The foramen magnum is outlined at A. The amount of herniation of the tonsils (B) is measured from the foramen magnum line.

The true cause of Chiari I malformation is unknown. As previously mentioned, it is considered a malformation that persons are born with. The reason that many people do not develop symptoms from the Chiari I malformation until their third or fourth decade of life is unknown. The malformation occurs more often in women than men (approximately 3:1), and in no particular ethnic or geographic distribution. Chiari I malformation can occur in both children and adults. Although infrequent, the Chiari I malformation may also be present in infancy, however the Chiari II malformation is more common in this age group. The true incidence in the general population is unknown. There is some information that the Chiari I malformation can run in some families and research is currently being performed in this area. The Type I malformation may also be associated with other structural abnormalities of the skull or cervical spine.

Chiari Type II malformation is generally diagnosed in infants and children. It is characterized by elongation of the cerebellar and posterior fossa structures. The fourth ventricle and portion of the brainstem may also be displaced through the foramen magnum into the upper cervical canal. Type II is nearly always associated with myelomeningocele, or spina bifida aperta. This type of hindbrain herniation also includes a smaller than normal posterior fossa. Chiari type II carries a higher incidence of morbidity and mortality than the type I malformation. The infant with an open neural tube defect (or myelomeningocele) is often diagnosed while the mother is pregnant using ultrasound, or immediately after birth. In most cases, the myelomeningocele is surgically repaired within 24-36 hours after birth. However, the Chiari type II may not be symptomatic until later in infancy or childhood, and some people never develop symptoms.

Chiari Type III malformation is a rare disorder that is characterized by a cervical fluid filled sac (meningocele) that may contain portions of the posterior fossa structures. The type III Chiari malformation is diagnosed in infancy and carries a cautious prognosis.

Some people can develop the Chiari malformation due to causes such as lumbar shunt, repeated lumbar punctures, or mass lesions within the brain that pull or push the cerebellar tonsils downward. Such mass lesions can include cyst or tumor. The treatment of acquired tonsillar herniation depends on the cause.

About one-fourth to one-half of persons with the Chiari I malformation are found to have other associated congenital abnormalities of the bones at the base of the skull or upper neck. These abnormalities can also be found in individuals who do not have Chiari malformation and usually do not cause symptoms. These abnormalities occur during fetal development and include the following:

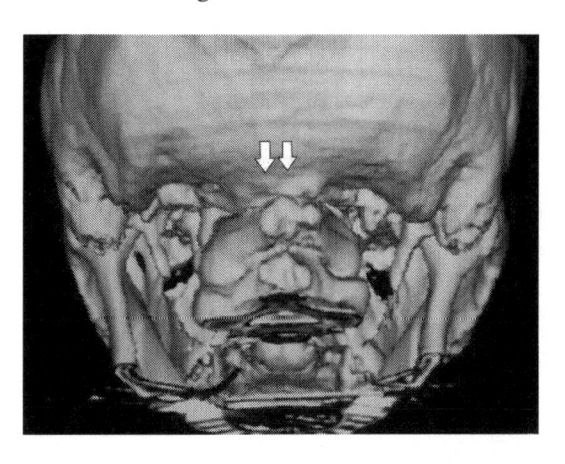

Assimilation of the atlas (C1) (above) — The first cervical vertebrae, called C1, is congenitally fused to the bottom of the skull at the foramen magnum.

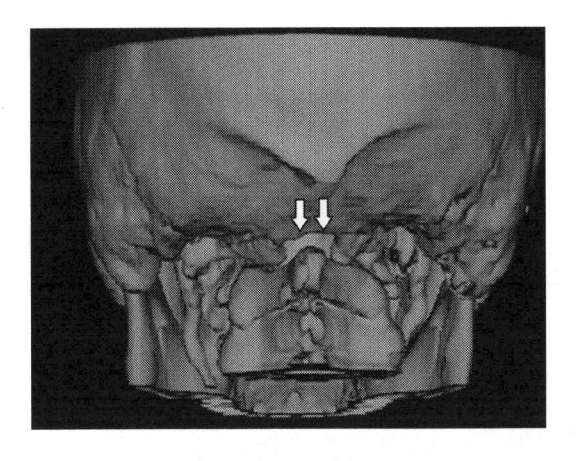

Bifid C1 lamina (above) — This is an image of a reconstructed CT scan of the back of the skull and the upper cervical spine. The back part of each spinal vertebra is called the *lamina*. It forms a roof over the spinal canal. When the C1 lamina is not completely formed and has a gap in it, it is known as a bifid lamina. This generally does not show on x-ray images, but can easily be seen on a CT scan. The bifid lamina does not cause symptoms.

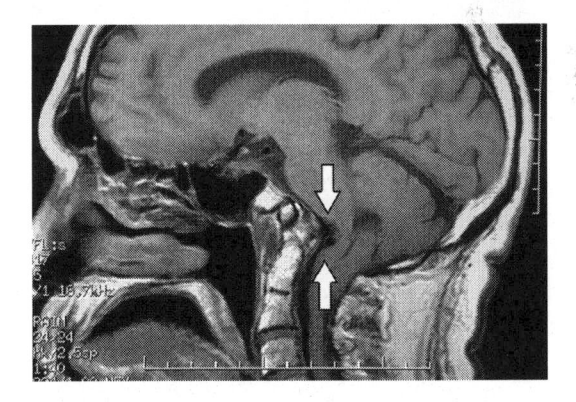

Basilar Impression (above) — The bone of the skull base around the foramen magnum and the upper cervical vertebrae are displaced up into the posterior fossa and result in indentation or kinking of the brainstem.

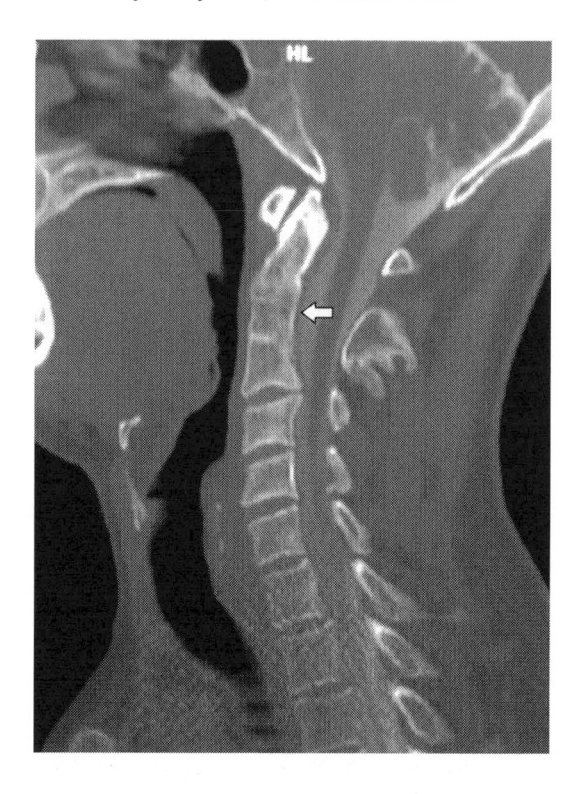

Klipple-Feil deformity (above)—This bone deformity was originally described by Dr Klippel and Dr. Feil in 1912. Characteristics include congenital fusion of two or more cervical vertebrae, with absent disc space and smaller than normal foramina, lower than normal hairline, short neck and, in most cases, restriction of the range of motion of the neck. On case above, the CT-myelogram of the cervical spine shows fusion of cervical 2, 3 & 4 vertebra.

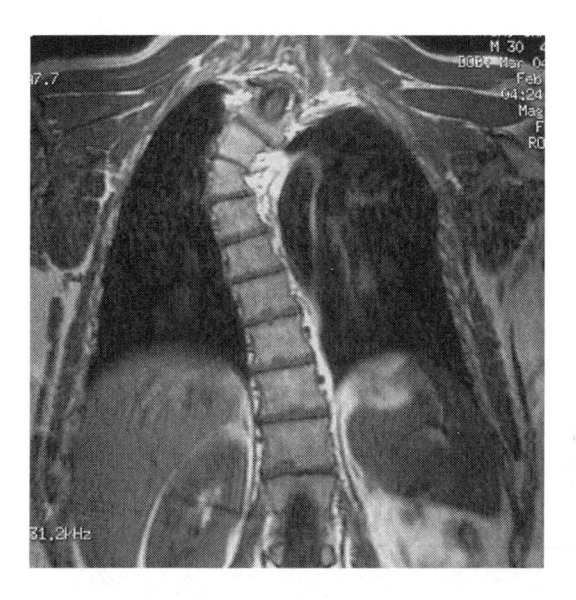

Scoliosis (above) — Scoliosis is a deformity of the spinal vertebrae that results in abnormal curvature of the spine. In patients with Chiari I malformation, this is most often associated with syringomyelia. The image above is an MRI of the thoracic spine showing scoliosis.

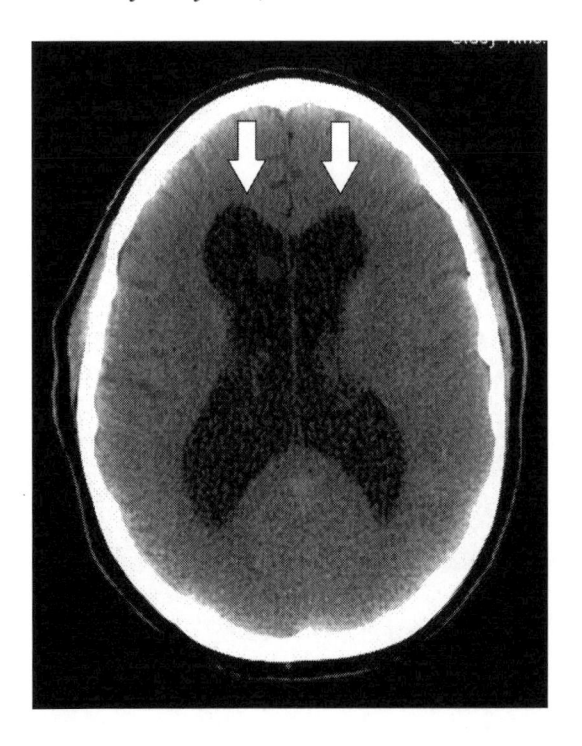

Hydrocephalus (above)—Although not a bony deformity of the skull or cervical spine, the Chiari I malformation can sometimes be associated with hydrocephalus. The MRI above shows enlargement of the ventricles in a person with hydrocephalus.

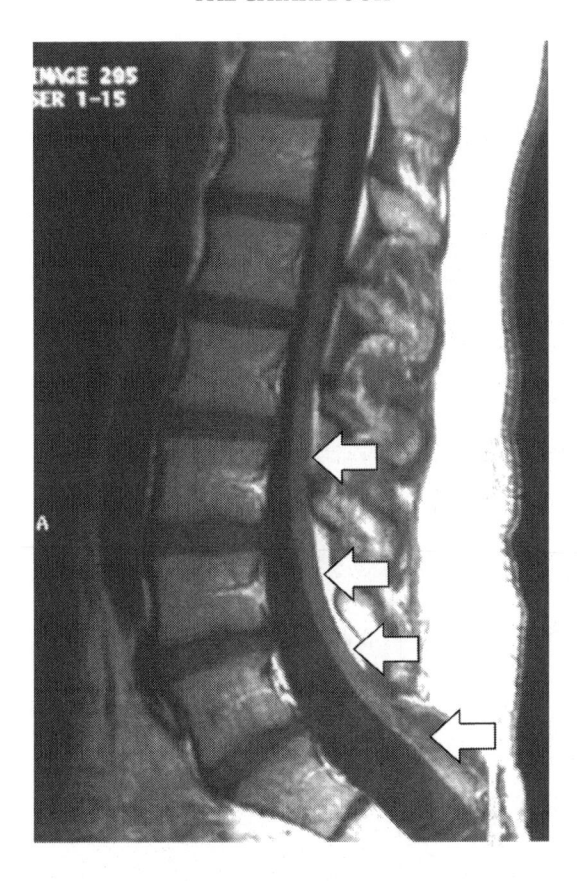

Spina Bifida Occulta, or tethered cord is most often associated with Chiari type II malformation. The lower part of the spinal cord is in an abnormally low position and is tethered in the sacral region by a thick filum (The filum is normally a thin cord at the end of the spinal cord) or a mass, usually a lipoma (fatty tumor). The MRI of the lumbar spine above shows the spinal cord extending all the way down the spinal canal in a 22-year-old patient with the Chiari type II malformation (not shown).

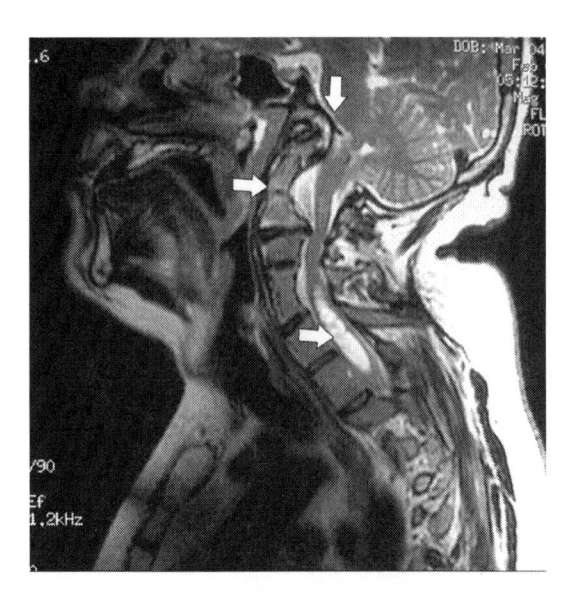

Multiple malformations (above)—Some persons can have multiple abnormalities that can either be symptomatic or asymptomatic. The above image shows a cervical MRI of a person with multiple abnormalities, including Klippel-Feil deformity, basilar invagination, cervical kyphoscoliosis, Chiari I malformation and cervical syringomyelia

CHAPTER 4

SYRINGOMYELIA

The brainstem joins the spinal cord at the foramen magnum located at the bottom of the skull. The spinal cord is a long, thin, delicate structure that rests within the *spinal canal*. The spinal canal is a tubular space that allows the flow of cerebrospinal fluid (CSF) around the spinal cord. The spinal canal is made of two coverings: the *dura* and the *arachnoid* membrane. The dura is the tough outer covering and the arachnoid is the thin transparent membrane just inside the dura. The arachnoid is filled with spinal fluid and contains the spinal cord. Normally, the spinal cord ends at about the first or second lumbar vertebra in the adult. The spinal canal is surrounded and protected by the bony structure of the spinal column (or vertebra).

The cerebrospinal fluid surrounds the spinal cord and travels from the brain, down the spinal canal and back up to the intracranial cavity. Normally, there is no CSF collection within the spinal cord, instead, the fluid surrounds the cord. The function of the CSF is to bathe and protect the brain and spinal cord. Many nerves originate from the spinal cord, and are responsible for movement and sensation of the arms, legs and the torso.

Syringomyelia (sir-ing-o-my-eel-ya) was first described by Antoine Portal in 1803. He described a patient who experienced numbness and loss of function of the lower extremities. An examination after death of the patient found a cavity, called a syrinx (see-rin-x), in the spinal cord. The condition is known as Syringomyelia and is defined as an abnormal fluid cavity (something like a long blister) inside the spinal cord. Spinal fluid should be in the spinal canal and outside of the spinal cord, not inside the spinal cord. If spinal fluid collects inside the spinal cord, it creates a syrinx that causes pressure and disruption of the normal function of the nerves that travel in that area of the cord. In most cases of syringomyelia due to the Chiari I malformation, the syrinx occurs in the area of the cervical spine. It may extend down into the spinal cord in the thoracic spine. In a few patients, it may just be present in the thoracic spine. Some people can have extensive syringomyelia (called holocord syringomyelia) that extends from the upper cervical spine down to the end of the spinal cord in the upper part of the lumbar spine.

One of the most famous persons of the past century who suffered from syringomyelia was Robert Tyre Jones, more commonly known as Bobby Jones. Born in Atlanta, Georgia in 1902, Bobby Jones is best known for winning the Grand Slam of golf in 1930 at the age of 29. He is responsible for designing the first set of matched golf clubs to be mass-produced and was the first to use numbers on the clubs instead of Scottish names. Bobby Jones established the Masters Tournament, which remains one of the most prestigious golf tournaments in the world. In the middle of his career, he played in considerable pain until he was diagnosed with syringomyelia in 1956. His neurological function continued to deteriorate until his death in 1971 at the age of 69. In his later life, when asked how he coped with his illness after being such a stellar sports figure, he simply said, "Remember, we play the ball as it lies." Fortunately today, with advances in diagnosis and treatment, the progression of syringomyelia can often be arrested.

The most common cause of syringomyelia is the Chiari I Malformation. Theories suggest that if a Chiari malformation is left untreated, a syrinx may form over time. However, not everyone with the Chiari malformation will develop a syrinx. Other causes of syringomyelia include trauma to the spinal cord, spinal cord tumors, or *arachnoiditis* (inflammation of the arachnoid layer of the covering of the spinal cord). Some people have syringomyelia without any identifiable cause: this is called *idiopathic* (unknown cause) syringomyelia. Although the exact mechanism of development of syringomyelia is unknown, there are many theories about the formation of a syrinx cavity. One theory suggests that the herniated tonsils such as in the Chiari I Malformation, result in blockage at the funnel at the base of the skull that connects to the spinal canal. This changes the fluid pressure around the spinal cord and causes fluid to accumulate in the spinal cord tissue. With each heartbeat, the spinal fluid pulsates. Therefore each pulsation forces fluid down the abnormal pathway. The syrinx (or fluid cavity) can enlarge over time, and puts pressure on the delicate nerve fibers within the spinal cord. There is no predictable pattern of enlargement of the syrinx cavity. Some will stay unchanged for years, while others may enlarge over months. Fortunately, those that enlarge, most often do so slowly.

The test of choice for diagnosis of syringomyelia is an MRI of the spine. The MRI may include the intravenous injection of contrast dye to determine if there is an associated tumor or inflammation of the arachnoid membrane (arachnoiditis). The most common place for a syrinx to develop is in the cervical spine, with the second most common in the thoracic spine. As the syrinx grows in size, it may cause scoliosis (abnormal curvature of the spine), which is best determined on x-ray of the spine.

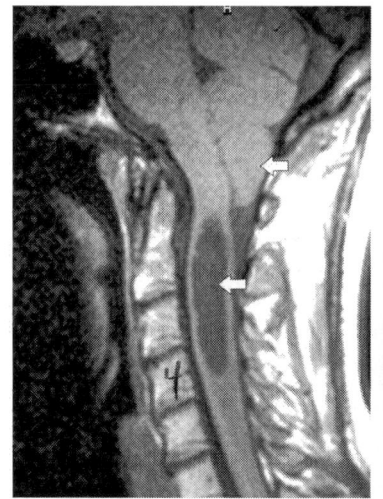

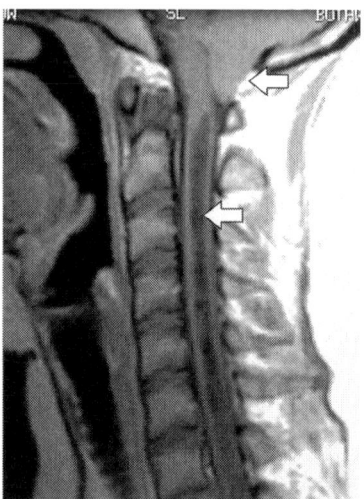

Images 1 and 2 (above)- side-view MRI scans of the cervical spine showing cervical syringomyelia and Chiari I malformation.

Many of the symptoms of syringomyelia are vague and variable, however symptoms can be progressive over a long period of time. If left untreated, long-standing stress on the spinal cord tissue can lead to permanent neurologic damage.

Pain is one of the most common symptoms persons report. In most cases, pain is located in the area of the body supplied by the nerves around the syrinx. For example, a person who has a thoracic syrinx may complain of pain in the mid-back or between the shoulder blades, or traveling from the back to below the ribs. Some people report pain in the arm, hand or leg. The pain is most often described as burning in nature, but can also be described as dull and aching, or stabbing. Pain in the extremities on one side (unilateral) is more commonly reported than on both sides (bilateral).

Paresthesias and numbness- Some people report tingling pins and needles sensation (called *paresthesia*) or numbness in the back or extremities. Some report numbness to the point of burning or injuring themselves without realizing the extent of the injury. Numbness can radiate from the back to below the ribs or the flank. Many people think they are having a heart attack because of sudden tingling in the arm. If this happens, it is best to seek medical attention immediately to rule out a heart attack. Persons can have pain, numbness and tingling in the extremity at the same time.

The treatment of syringomyelia is discussed in Chapter 8.

CHAPTER 5

SYMPTOMS OF THE CHIARI I MALFORMATION

The early symptoms of Chiari I malformation (CMI) may be vague, transient and variable. The degrees of symptoms present in CMI do not necessarily correlate with the amount of tonsillar herniation as represented on MRI. For example, one person with tonsillar herniation of 5mm on MRI can have severe, debilitating symptoms, while another can have very mild symptoms and over 15mm tonsillar herniation on MRI. Often the symptoms are present for months or years, and in some cases, are reported as long as the patient can recall. Many adult patients report symptoms, particularly headache, as far back as elementary school. Symptoms may vary in severity and can be inactive or stable for months to years. Some persons will report symptoms being triggered by an injury, such as motor vehicle crash, whiplash, roller coaster ride, or minor injury to the head or neck. Most of the symptoms of Chiari I malformation can be attributed to obstruction of the flow of CSF, or compression of the lower brainstem and cranial nerves. Common presenting symptoms include:

- ***Headache*** is the most common presenting symptom and is reported by up to 98% of individuals with Chiari I malformation. The pain usually starts in the occipital region (back of the skull), and radiates to the top of the head, or behind the eyes or temporal areas. It is most often triggered by activities such as coughing, straining, laughing, bending or lifting. The pain is often described as pressure and can also be explosive, dull, aching, vice-like or band-like in nature. It usually varies in severity from mild to unbearable. The head pain can last for hours to days, or it can be constant. Severe head pain may be associated with nausea and/or vomiting, but rarely vomiting without nausea.

- *Dizziness* is one of the most common symptoms reported by patients. A feeling of light-headedness, or floating is the most common description. Dizziness occurs intermittently, and is often made worse by quick movements, or worsened by lying flat. Vertigo (intense spinning) is less common.

- *Disequilibrium* (poor balance) is a very troubling symptom for many people, and some report difficulty with stairs, or uneven ground. Patients may report falling or bumping into walls or furniture. Some persons resort to the use of assistive devices for ambulation (walking).

- *Pain* of varying degrees is one of the most common presenting symptoms. Pain can occur in the neck, face, jaw, arms and legs, or back. Neck pain is the most common type of pain and may result in limited range of movement of the cervical spine. Pain in one arm or leg is reported more often than in both, arms or legs. The pain can be described as aching, sharp, or stabbing in nature. Arm pain is more common than leg pain. Pain in the chest area that is described as *'burning'* in nature may be due to syringomyelia.

- *Numbness, tingling, or pins-and-needles sensations in the arm or leg* are frequently reported and can be associated with weakness. These sensory disturbances generally occur on one side, but can progress to both sides, upper and lower extremities, and the trunk. Fine motor skills, such as buttoning buttons, can be negatively affected. In the presence of untreated syringomyelia, numbness can progress to partial weakness or even paralysis in advanced cases. Numbness can also be reported in the face now and then, and is often worse with severe headache.

- ***Difficulty Swallowing (dysphagia),*** which may be the result of compression of the lower cranial nerves is generally described as a 'catch in the throat' or a feeling of mechanical swallowing difficulty. Some persons report choking on either liquids or solids. Dysphagia may progress from simple complaints of difficulty swallowing to frank aspiration of food and fluids. Difficulty swallowing saliva or choking sensation while lying flat is commonly reported.

- ***Weakness of the extremities*** is more common in the arms than the legs. Weakness on one side is more common than weakness on both sides. However, some persons will report diffuse, generalized body weakness. Weakness may be progressive over time, generally in an ascending (bottom-to-top) pattern. Clumsiness or weakness of the hand(s) and difficulty with fine motor skills is generally reported prior to weakness of the feet or legs.

- ***Neuro-ophthalomogic symptoms*** can be somewhat vague and short-lived. Visual changes can range from occasional blurred vision, to diplopia (double vision), to visual field cuts. Transient, unilateral vision loss is uncommon, but has been reported. Many patients described tunnel vision or seeing "spots" in the periphery. *Nystagmus* (bobbing of the eyes) or rotatory nystagmus is not uncommon. *Photophobia,* or sensitivity to light, is also commonly reported, and some people feel they require dark glasses at all times.

- ***Neuro-otologic symptoms*** include unilateral or bilateral ringing in the ears (*tinnitus*), hearing loss or abnormal sounds. Abnormal sounds can be described as chirping, buzzing or a 'whooshing' sound. Decreased hearing is also common, with both ears being affected. Persons often reported inability to hear while on the telephone or when extraneous noise is present. Ear ache/pressure is less common, but can occur.

- ***Shortness of breath*** unrelated to exertion is frequently reported. This is can become worse when lying flat, and may disrupt sleep patterns. *Sleep apnea,* which should be confirmed by formal sleep testing, may occur, and some persons require CPAP (continuous positive airway pressure) at night. CPAP is a device that delivers positive airway pressure that helps breathing. The patient's spouse or significant other may also report a significant increase in the volume and frequency of snoring while asleep.

- ***Difficulty sleeping-*** Patients frequently report difficulty sleeping due to pain, anxiety, difficulty breathing when lying down, or generalized insomnia. Patients also report increased sleepiness, and the desire to sleep more than 10 hours per day. Most persons who note difficulty sleeping, report feeling "tired all the time". Generalized fatigue is very common in patients with Chiari malformation. Patients can describe non-refreshing sleep, although they had slept over 8 hours per night. Lack of restful sleep may result in a significant impact on the patient's ability to perform daily activities or cognitive function due to fatigue and exhaustion

- ***Speech difficulty***, including slurred speech and word finding problems, are very common among those with Chiari malformation. *Hoarseness,* raspiness, or change in the quality or timbre of the voice, is also very common. Many patients state they are unable to sing due to inability to modulate their voice.

- ***Nausea*** is much more frequently reported than *vomiting*. Patients experience nausea, in correlation with head pain. Increased nausea is also more frequently noted during episodes of dizziness. Abdominal pain, indigestion, constipation, and change in appetite are also frequently reported.

- ***Memory Problems*** are a frequent concern for individuals with Chiari malformation. Memory difficulty ranges from simple forgetfulness to difficulty with concentration, or more serious reports by family members of safety concerns. Some persons will report a feeling of 'being in a fog". Concentration difficulty can affect the individual's ability to perform job related tasks or undertake new responsibilities.

- ***Depression, anxiety*** and a feeling of hopelessness are very commonly reported among persons with Chiari I malformation. The depression may result from the situation the person finds themselves due to pain, difficulty sleeping, and chronic illness. Thoughts of suicide are reported by a few persons, and should be evaluated by a trained counselor.

- ***Cardiac symptoms*** can include chest pain, episodic tachycardia and palpitations. Cardiac arrhythmias are not generally reported among persons with Chiari malformation, and should be evaluated by a cardiologist. Persons who complain of persistent burning type pain radiating from the mid-back around the front to below the ribs or sternum should be suspicious for syringomyelia. It is best to have an evaluation by a cardiologist to rule out any heart related problems.

CHAPTER 6

OTHER ILLNESSES THAT CAN MIMIC CHIARI MALFORMATION

As discussed in Chapter 5, the symptoms of Chiari I malformation can be vague, transient, and often *insidious* (developing so slowly that they may at first not be noticed). Many other neurologic and metabolic disorders can result in symptoms that mimic (act-like) those of CMI. It is also important to remember that not all symptoms are likely due to Chiari I malformation, and a person can have several unrelated disorders. When being evaluated for the possibility of Chiari malformation, it is important that other medical conditions be considered as a possible cause of the symptoms. Often, evaluation may take a team of specialists to determine causes. The evaluation team may include a neurosurgeon, neurologist, ear nose and throat specialist, neuro-ophthalmologist, cardiologist, internist, pain specialist, specially trained nurses, physiatrist, psychiatrist and neuropsychologist. Some disorders are diagnosed with blood tests, MRI, or other diagnostic tests while others are more difficult to diagnose.

Among the conditions that can mimic the CMI are:

Ataxia- Gait imbalance can be due to many causes. Some of the more common conditions include metabolic disorders, such as hypo/hyperthyroid, vitamin deficiency, dietary deficiency, anemia, medication toxicity, lead poisoning, environmental toxin exposure, alcoholism, polypharmacy or medication interactions. Disorders of the brain can include stroke, brain tumor (particularly cerebellar tumors), arachnoid cyst involving the cerebellum, encephalopathy, cerebellar atrophy, multiple sclerosis, cerebellar abscess, and brain trauma/injury. Disorders not related to the brain tissue include diabetic neuropathy, polyneuropathy, and post-polio syndrome. Disorders of the cervical or thoracic spine can also cause gait disturbances. These include degenerative discs, spinal canal narrowing (stenosis), syringomyelia, multiple sclerosis, and tumors of the spine or spinal cord.

Blurred vision and/or double vision (diplopia) can be caused by problems of the eye itself, or disorders within the brain. Uncontrolled hypertension can cause visual problems and can often be controlled with medication. Ocular problems are best evaluated by a neuro-ophthalmologist, and may include orbital infections, retinal detachment, myosis, or ocular nerve lesions. Systemic conditions to be considered include hypertension, hypo/hyperthyroid, diabetes, botulism, lead poisoning, vitamin disorders, multiple medication regimen (polypharmacy), alcoholism, medication toxicity, and medication interactions. Disorders of the nervous system that can cause blurred vision or double vision include Multiple Sclerosis, Myasthenia Gravis, pituitary lesions, brain tumor, encephalitis, brain abscess, and migraine with aura.

Cognitive problems can vary from simple memory difficulty to severe cognitive impairment, and often requires evaluation with formal testing by a trained neuropsychologist. Systemic causes of mental status changes include medication toxicity, medication interactions, substance abuse, alcoholism, severe depression, chronic pain, exposure to environmental toxins, vitamin deficiency, anemia, infections, nutritional deficiency, thyroid imbalance, and metabolic imbalance. Brainstem disorders that can cause cognitive problems include brain tumors (particularly of the frontal lobe), multiple sclerosis, vascular insufficiency, brain injury, brain abscess, and stroke.

Other causes include Parkinson's disease, Alzheimer's disease, multi-infarct state, Pick's disease, and other neurodegenerative disorders.

Dizziness and vertigo can be difficult to assess due to the many factors that can cause these symptoms. The evaluation often involves a variety of specialists including a neurologist, ear nose and throat specialist (ENT), neuro-ophthalmologist, psychiatrist and neurosurgeon. Systemic causes of dizziness and vertigo include anemia, cardiac arrhythmias, hypertension, hypotension, medication toxicity, polypharmacy, alcohol or substance abuse, heavy metal exposure, infections, pulmonary insufficiency, diabetes, hyper/hypothyroidism, and hypoglycemia. Disorders related to the inner ear can often result in vertigo, and can include labyrinthitis, vestibular neuritis, mass lesions of the vestibular nerve, and inner ear infections. Brain abnormalities that can cause dizziness or vertigo include vascular insufficiency, carotid artery stenosis, stroke, transient ischemic attacks (TIA), multiple sclerosis, tumor, infections, abscess, seizures, encephalopathy, brain injury and post-concussion syndrome. Dizziness and vertigo may also be due to neuropsychological disorders such as anxiety, panic disorder, vasovagal response, hyperventilation syndrome, and non-epileptic seizures.

Dysphagia, or difficulty swallowing, can signify a disorder of the mechanism of swallowing, or can result from compression on the cranial nerve that controls the ability to swallow. Disorders of the esophagus that can cause dysphagia include esophagitis, cancers of the mouth or throat, hiatal hernia, gastric reflux, pharyngitis, diverticulum, or esophageal spasm. Systemic causes include metabolic disorders, heavy metal exposure, Lupus, and vitamin deficiency. Neurologic causes include tumor, Myasthenia Gravis, Multiple Sclerosis, basilar invagination, and ALS (amyotrophic lateral sclerosis or Lou Gehrig's disease).

Extremity weakness, pain and paresthesia can be vague and episodic, and can occur on one side (unilateral) or both sides (bilateral). Systemic causes include fibromyalgia, chronic fatigue syndrome, metabolic disorders, thyroid disorder, renal insufficiency, vitamin deficiency, polypharmacy, hypertension, Lyme disease, post-polio syndrome, renal disorders, heavy metal exposure, or Lupus. Central nervous system disorders include Multiple Sclerosis, Myasthenia Gravis, ALS, neuropathy, brain or spine tumor, cervical spinal stenosis, syringomyelia, herniated cervical disc with spinal cord compression, or neurosarcoidosis.

Fatigue is one of the most vague and inconsistent complaints and can be associated with a myriad of disorders. Fatigue can occur to most people at some point in their life. However, relentless, intractable fatigue, or that which is associated with inability to function in daily life is a more serious concern. The systemic causes of fatigue are too numerous to list, but include anemia, vitamin deficiency, metabolic disorders, thyroid imbalance, renal imbalance, chronic fatigue syndrome, pulmonary insufficiency, cardiac deficiency, Lupus, Hepatitis, liver disease, substance abuse, heavy metal exposure, insomnia, sleep apnea and severe depression. The neurologic causes of incapacitating fatigue include Multiple Sclerosis, Myasthenia Gravis, brain tumor, brain infection, ALS, post-polio syndrome, pituitary lesion, and central sleep apnea.

Headache is the most common symptom reported among persons with Chiari malformation. However, it is important to remember that headache is a symptom, and can be attributed to many other disorders. Primary headache disorders can include migraine, cluster headache, tension, post concussion syndrome and vascular headache. Pseudotumor cerebri is a condition of sustained intracranial hypertension, without an actual tumor that can cause persistent headaches. Disorders of the head and neck, which can result in headache, may include temporomandibular joint disorder (TMJ), disease of the teeth or gums, temporal arteritis, occipital neuralgia, trigeminal neuralgia, cervical strain and spasm, cervical stenosis, and basilar invagination. Ocular (eye) disorders, such as glaucoma, and eye strain can cause headache. Sinusitis, allergies, and sinus congestion are some of the most common causes of headache. Systemic causes of headache can include hypertension, medication rebound, polypharmacy, alcohol or substance abuse, caffeinism, insomnia, tobacco use, stress, depression, vitamin deficiency, metabolic disorders, Lyme disease and infections. Headaches associated with problems within the brain include tumors, arachnoid cyst, abscess, infections, vascular malformation, aneurysm, vascular spasm, trauma, and a blood clot in the brain.

Hearing loss and/ or tinnitus is a symptom that can be due to problems within the ear itself or within the brain. The common ear-related problems include cerumen (ear wax) impaction, tumor within the ear, myringitis, labyrinthitis, Meniere's disease, membrane perforation, infections, excessive noise injury to the ear, and foreign objects in the ear canal. Familial hearing loss can be a family related trait, and can lead to hearing loss at a young age. Tinnitus (ringing in the ears) can be due to infection, tumor of the vestibular nerve, cyst, or otitis. Systemic disorders that can cause hearing loss or tinnitus include diabetes, mumps, vitamin toxicity, medication toxicity (particularly aspirin), hypo/hyperthyroidism, allergies, sinusitis, or viral infections. Intracranial problems can include tumor, or infection.

Hoarseness or voice changes can be due to mechanical problems, such as esophageal tumor, vocal cord paralysis, vocal cord polyps, laryngitis, esophagitis, basilar invagination, or throat trauma. Systemic causes can include vitamin deficiency, nutritional deficiency, tobacco use, inhalation of toxins or environmental exposure, iodine deficiency, anxiety or panic attacks. Compression of the cranial nerves from tumor or expanding mass lesion can also result in voice changes.

CHAPTER 7

THE DIAGNOSIS OF CHIARI MALFORMATION AND SYRINGOMYELIA

The Neurological Examination

After obtaining a thorough medical history, including the past medical/surgical history, vital signs, weight, medication history and family/social history, the next step in the evaluation is a thorough neurologic examination. This is one of the most important pieces of the diagnostic process. Although some persons with radiographic evidence of Chiari I malformation on MRI will have a completely normal examination, some people will have important abnormal findings (or deficits).

All or some of the following test(s) may be done during the clinic visit.

- *Cognitive evaluation (thinking processes)*- The patient may be asked such questions as the date, place, and the patient's full name. This helps to determine if there is a problem with thinking and memory. It is important that the patient does not get any help from family/friends during this evaluation. The patient may be asked to recite a common phrase or write a sentence. This helps to assess any speech problems. Abnormal speech may be called dysarthria.

- ***Cranial nerves*** - There are 12 cranial nerves that help to control many movements and sensations throughout the head and upper neck. There are nerves within the brain that control facial movements and sensation. Eye movements are checked by asking the patient to follow the examiner's finger in several different directions. Shining a light in each eye determines if the pupils react properly. The back of the eye is examined with a special light (see *Fundoscopic examination* below). Facial sensation is checked by lightly stroking the face with the fingers or a Q-tip to determine if there is any area of decreased or abnormal sensation. Facial muscles are checked by asking the patient to smile, grimace, and close their eyes tightly. Hearing is checked by the examiner lightly rubbing their fingers together in close proximity to the ears to see if there is any subjective decreased hearing. Movement of the tongue is checked by having the patient stick out the tongue and move from side to side. Uneven movement of the tongue and palate are important cranial nerve functions as well. Taste and smell are sometimes checked in the clinic. The gag reflex is checked with a tongue blade, lightly touching the back of the throat. A normal response would be to gag. Absence of gag response may be due to compression of the nerve that controls this reflex. The patient may be asked to shrug their shoulders, and move their head from side to side, as this is also controlled by the cranial nerves.

- ***Fundoscopic examination*** — The fundus is the back of the eye and can be seen by looking through the pupil. The test is performed using a special instrument called an ophthalmoscope. With the bright light of the ophthalmoscope, the examiner can look at the optic nerve and the blood vessels on the retina, and look for signs of nerve swelling, hemorrhage or other abnormalities. This is a painless test, but the patient should alert the examiner if they are particularly sensitive to bright light. If the optic nerve or blood vessels are found to be abnormal, a referral to an ophthalmologist or a neuro-ophthalmologist (special eye doctor who is a expert in both ophthalmology and neuroscience) may be requested.

- *Motor examination*- The motor examination tests strength in the arms and legs. This is generally done by testing handgrips, arm strength, and leg strength. The patient will be asked to grip the fingers of the examiner to test hand grip strength. Biceps, triceps and deltoid muscles are tested by having the patient resist the push/pull of the examiner. Lower extremity strength is tested in the same fashion by having the patient push/pull against the examiner. It is helpful to give this test all effort possible, as strength is an important component of the examination. Holding both arms outward with the palms up and both eyes closed tests abnormal movement of the extremities. Inability to maintain both arms out is called pronator drift.

- *Sensory examination*- Sensory testing will help to determine if there are any areas with numbness or decreased sensation. This test is done on several areas of the body. The face is lightly stroked with the fingers or a Q-tip by the examiner to determine if there is any numbness or tingling. The upper and lower extremities are lightly stroked with the fingers, and then tested by light pinprick to determine if there is any decrease in sensation, numbness or tingling. If a patient reports numbness or tingling in the upper back, this area may be tested as well. Vibration sense is tested with a tuning fork.

- **Reflexes-** The test is done to determine if the reflexes react normally to a stimulus. A small reflex hammer is used to tap the arms, knees and ankles. The reflexes should normally "jump" when tapped. Some people have absent reflexes, which may be normal in their specific case. For example, some athletes will have decreased reflexes in the knees- this may be normal for them. The most important abnormal finding is very brisk reflexes, crossed reflexes (reflexes that spread to the opposite side), or any asymmetry between the sides being tested. This may signify compression on the spinal cord.

- **Cerebellar function-** Because the cerebellum is the area of the brain that controls coordination of movement, tests will be done to determine if this area is functioning properly. Many persons with the Chiari I malformation can have problems with cerebellar functions, and report imbalance. The patient may be asked to walk both normally and in a straight line to observe any gait imbalance. If a person is unable to walk a straight line, this is called *gait ataxia*. The patient will be asked to touch his/her index finger to their nose, back to the finger of the examiner, and back and forth quickly. This tests any inability to coordinate movement of the hands, which is called *dysmetria*. Rapid alternating movements are tested by quickly turning the hand back and forth (pronation/supination) while resting on the thigh. A test, called the *Romberg* test, is performed by standing with both eyes closed and feet together, while trying to keep an erect posture. This tests balance.

Radiological Studies

Magnetic resonance imaging (MRI) gives detailed pictures of the brain, the spinal cord, and the surrounding tissues. The MRI (sometimes including the injection of a contrast material into a vein) is used to diagnose tumors, hydrocephalus, intracranial blood, and other abnormalities. When people without neurological symptoms undergo an MRI of the brain, the tonsils are usually found to be an average of 0-3 mm <u>above</u> the foramen magnum, whereas those with Chiari will usually have tonsils 3-5 mm or more <u>below</u> the foramen magnum (image below).

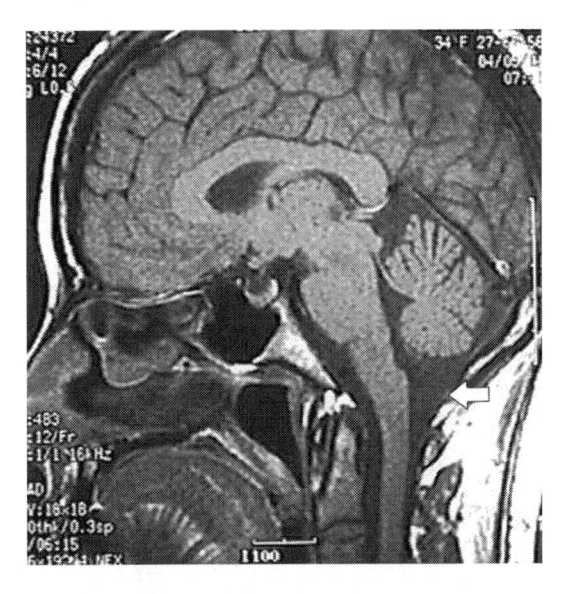

Image 1: A normal side-view MRI scan. The area at the foramen magnum is open and there is no crowding of the tissues.

The radiographic test of choice to diagnose the Chiari I malformation is the MRI (magnetic resonance imaging) of the brain. For the purpose of diagnosing Chiari malformation, this test generally does not require injection of contrast dye. An MRI is a test using a large magnet to obtain pictures (called *images*) instead of x-rays. The MRI images will show if there is crowding at the opening of the bottom of the skull, known as the foramen magnum. The test is performed by having the person lie on a flat imaging table that slides into an enclosed tube. It is important to lie very still while in the scanner, as the pictures are very sensitive to movement. There is a machine-like sound while the pictures are taken. The space inside the tube is quite snug, therefore, be sure to tell the technician or health care provider if there is any history of claustrophobia or being uncomfortable in small, tight places. Because the test is performed with a special high-power magnet, it may not be performed on anyone with a metal implant (such as artificial limbs, artificial metal joints, aneurysm clips, shrapnel, metal heart valves, or pacemakers). If the patient is unsure of any metal inside the body, the MRI technician should be notified before the test begins. Images 2 and 3 below are MRI scans showing the Chiari I malformation.

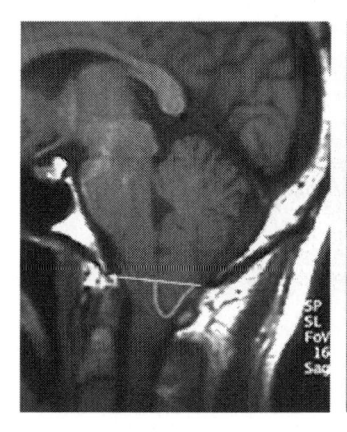

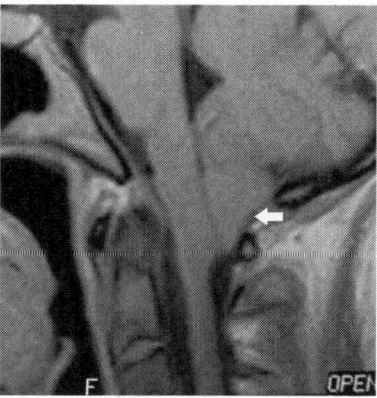

Images 2 & 3: These MRI scans are of two persons with the Chiari I malformation. The image on the left shows an imaginary line drawn across the foramen magnum. The cerebellar tonsils (outlined) are herniated below the line. On the MRI on the right, the cerebellar tonsils also hang down below the foramen magnum and crowd the cisterna magna, which is no longer visible.

The diagnosis of syringomyelia is confirmed with an MRI of the spine. Since there may be other causes of syringomyelia besides Chiari I malformation, an MRI with and without contrast dye may be requested to determine the presence of tumors or other abnormalities in the spine. The image that is most useful when diagnosing syringomyelia is the side-view (known as sagittal view) of the spine (Images 2 & 3).

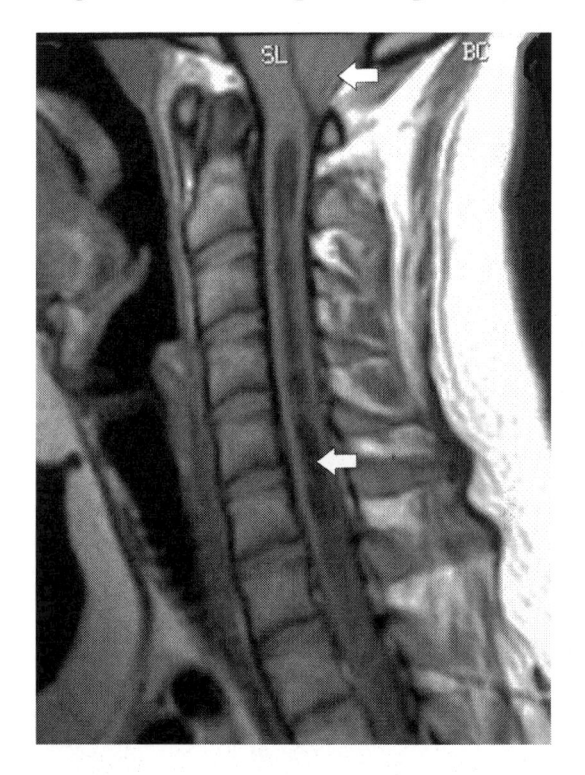

Figure 3: This side-view MRI of the cervical spine shows crowding at the foramen magnum due to a Chiari I malformation. The darker areas within the spinal cord are pockets of spinal fluid known as a syrinx or syringomyelia

A CSF flow study or CINE MRI is used to assess the flow of spinal fluid in the area of the foramen magnum. The test is done in the MRI scanner, in the same way as a regular MRI and looks at the flow of spinal fluid around the posterior fossa and the upper cervical spinal canal. The flow is generally observed during every pulse of the heart, and can be measured by a neuro-radiologist (radiologist trained in nervous system diagnosis).

X-rays of the neck- Over 50% of people with the Chiari I malformation also have some signs that the bones of the skull or spine did not develop properly. These are described in Chapter 3.

Persons with the Chiari I malformation can have other conditions of the neck that are <u>unrelated</u> to Chiari I. Some people can have a herniated cervical disc causing pain, numbness or tingling of the extremities. An MRI of the cervical spine can help to determine if this is causing the problem.

Cervical stenosis, a condition associated with age-related changes in the neck can also cause pain and numbness. In severe cases, stenosis can also cause weakness of the arms and legs, a condition called myelopathy.

Additional Studies

While not usually required, other studies may show abnormalities. Patients presenting with hearing loss or tinnitus may show abnormalities in specializes tests such as pure tone audiograms, auditory brain stem reflexes, and electronystagmography. Esophageal manometrics in patients with dysphagia (difficulty swallowing) may reveal markedly disordered esophageal motility and gastroesophageal reflux. Electromyography and nerve conduction tests may be helpful when the cause of weakness or numbness cannot be determined.

CHAPTER 8

TREATMENT OPTIONS FOR CHIARI MALFORMATION AND/OR SYRINGOMYELIA

The increasing use of MRI has resulted in more frequent recognition of patients with Chiari I malformation, many of whom do not have symptoms attributable to the malformation. These patients can be followed periodically with MRI of the cervical spine and surgical treatment can be reserved when unresponsive symptoms or evidence of syringomyelia develops.

Treatment options for patients with symptoms from the Chiari I malformation include non-operative (conservative) therapy and surgical intervention. Evaluation by a multidisciplinary team including a neurologist, a neurosurgeon, a physiatrist (rehabilitation physician), or other specialist may be necessary.

Non-operative or conservative therapy includes medications such as analgesics, anti-inflammatories, sedatives, antispasmotics and other newer headache medications. When neck pain or stiffness is a significant component, physical therapy may be of value. Physical therapy may include aerobic conditioning, cervical range of motion and strengthening, upper and lower trunk strengthening, abdominal strengthening, upper extremity and shoulder girdle strengthening and postural correction activities may aid in relief of back and extremity pain.

However, non-operative treatment in the presence of progressive symptoms frequently leads to chronic pain, often managed with narcotics. This may result in dependence and eventually may affect the patient's psychosocial function and decreases the likelihood of benefit from future surgical treatment should it be required.

Surgical treatment ranges from removal of bone at the back of the foramen magnum to extensive procedures that include placing a small piece of tissue at the bottom of the fourth ventricle in an area called the obex (now rarely performed). A consensus is developing among neurosurgeons who treat patients with Chiari I malformation for a moderate bony decompression followed by expansion of the dural sack with a tissue graft (duroplasty). Shrinkage of the tonsils (using a small operative instrument) in cases with marked crowding despite dural opening can play an important role in successful treatment. The treatment of choice for persons with symptoms associated with the Chiari I malformation, and who have failed to improve with non-surgical treatments, is surgery to decompress the posterior fossa area.

The main goal of surgical treatment for the Chiari malformation involves creating more space at the region of the foramen magnum to allow the spinal flow in this area to return to normal. This is a done by a procedure called **posterior fossa decompression**. At surgery, an incision is made at the back of the head that extends to the upper part of the neck. The muscles are spread to either side and the occipital bone and the back of the C1 vertebrae (the lamina) are visualized. Skull bone and the arch of C1 (in a few cases C2) are removed (Figure 1). The important point of the bone removal is to create enough of a bony decompression for spinal fluid to flow more normally and to avoid excessive bony decompression, which can result in cerebellar slump (Lack of support for part of the cerebellum, which then can partly slump into the upper spinal canal).

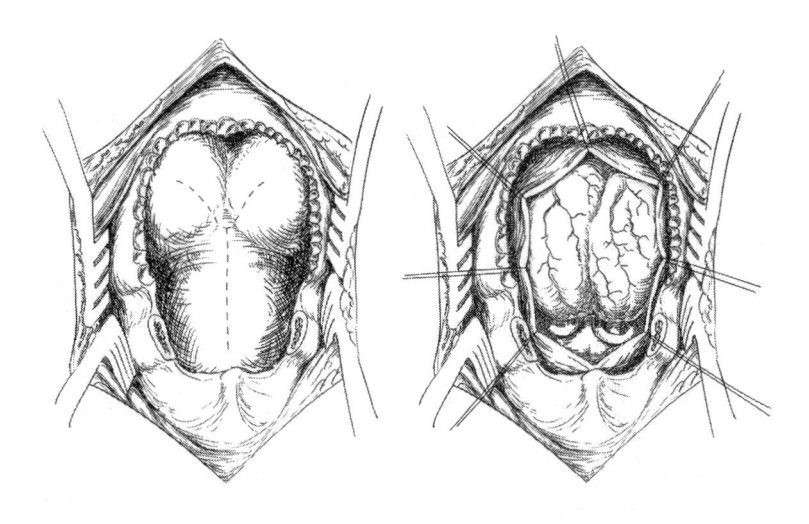

Figure 1: This view shows the area of the decompression surgery. The figure on the left shows the area of bone removal at the back of the skull and the removal of the back arch of the cervical 1 vertebrae. The membrane that is seen is the dura and will be opened in a Y-shaped fashion. The figure on the right shows the dura membrane open, the two tonsils, and below the tonsils, two of the blood vessels that go to the brain stem.

In infants and children, bony removal alone may be sufficient to provide the needed decompression. Studies are currently underway to help understand when this technique is most appropriate.

Under the bone is the tough membrane called the dura. The surgeon then opens the dura, usually with a Y-shaped incision, which results in a triangular shaped opening (Figure 1). If the crowding is not severe, the next layer- the transparent arachnoid- may not need to be opened. However, if there is a concern about fibrous bands within the arachnoid or the possibility that flow from the fourth ventricle (located between the brain stem and cerebellum) is not draining well into the cisterna magna, the arachnoid may be opened to release these bands and determine if there is a blockage of flow from the ventricle.

Some surgeons open the arachnoid and may shrink the tips of the tonsils with electrocautery. Studies to date do not indicate which procedure is best. There is no documented untoward effect from shrinking the tonsils. The surgical goal is to create more room so as to remove the crowding.

Most surgeons then sew a patch of material into the dura to enlarge the foramen magnum. Various patch materials can be used, including the patient's own tissue, (a lining on the surface of the skull called pericranium), bovine pericardium, or a synthetic material.

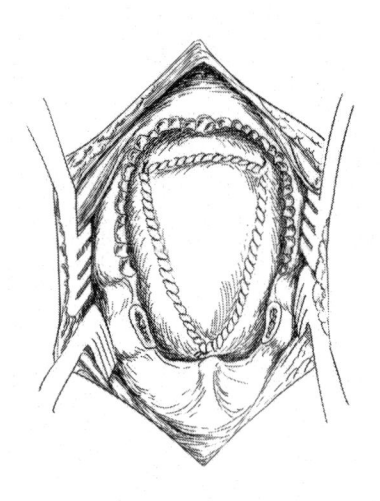

Figure 2: A pericranial graft has been obtained from underneath the scalp in the area above the decompression and sewn into the dural membrane to enlarge the area of the foramen magnum and the upper part of the spinal canal.

A recent addition to the surgical decompression procedure is the attachment of a small plate over a portion of the area of bone removal at the back of the skull (Figure 3). This is done in such a fashion as to avoid crowding of the area of decompression. The muscles that were previously attached to the bone in the area (now removed) can then be attached to the plate. This may lead to faster recovery of the muscles at the back of the neck.

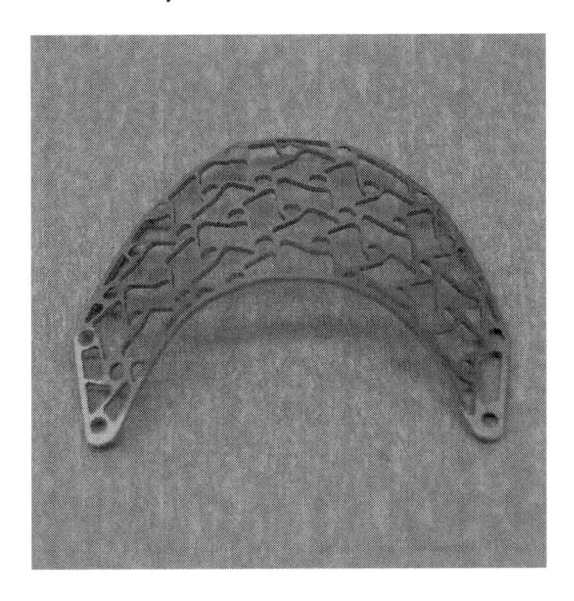

Figures 3: Plate for reconstruction of the skull after decompression for the Chiari I Malformation.

Closure of the wound is generally done with stitches to bring the muscles together and sutures or staples on the skin.

Outcome
The outcome following surgery for CMI is generally good. In 1989, Dyste, et al. presented the outcome in 50 patients with Chiari malformation, most having Chiari I. At follow-up, 20% were asymptomatic, 66% were improved, 8% were stabilized, and 6% showed progressive deterioration following surgical

treatment. More recent studies show an improved outcome. The reports of Hida in 1995 and Klekamp in 1996 reveal 77% to 97% of patients remain symptom free at 3- to 5-year follow-up. In a study by Mueller & Oro' (2005), detailed measurement of outcome one year following surgery revealed 84% of participants had significant improvement in their self-reported quality of life.

Many of the symptoms of Chiari I malformation respond to surgery. Cough headaches and cough syncope frequently resolve following posterior fossa decompression. Postoperative studies in patients with cough syncope show that the impaired control of heart rate to postural change returns to normal (Ireland 96). Follow-up studies in patients with disordered esophageal movement and gastroesophageal reflux can also return to normal following surgery (Elta 96). Weakness, however, is more difficult to treat and atrophy (loss of muscle tissue) rarely improves (Dyste 89).

Some patients will continue to have symptoms, progress or have a recurrence of symptoms despite surgical treatment. The factors that have the greatest negative impact on outcome include the presence of muscle atrophy and symptom duration of over 2 years (Dyste 89).

Risks

When making the decision to have surgery, the individual must weigh the quality of their life versus what is understood about the possible benefits and risks of surgery. There are certain risks to every operation. The operative risks of a posterior fossa decompression for the Chiari I malformation include (but are not limited to) bleeding from the operative site, wound infection, meningitis, spinal fluid leak and neurologic injury or stroke, postoperative neck pain or occipital neuralgia (a nerve pain at the back of the head). If the bony removal is too large, cerebellar slump can occur. The neurosurgeon should discuss the specific risks in detail with each individual patient prior to surgery.

Fortunately, serious neurological complications following surgery are rare. However, other complications can be troublesome. A p*seudomeningocele* is a collection of spinal fluid in the muscle tissues that results from a leak at the edge of the internal patch. Treatment usually requires lumbar drainage through a spinal catheter placed in the low back, or re-operation and closure of the site of the leak. Cerebellar slump, though rare, is treated by creation of more support using bone cement or a specialized plate.

What if I do nothing?

How an individual will do long term with symptoms from a Chiari I malformation is not known. If a person has symptoms that are intermittent (they come and go), and the MRI shows that there is no syrinx in the spinal cord, it is best to just watch and treat the headache with mild analgesics, physical therapy or headache medications. If symptoms are persistent and progressive, and haven't responded to conservative treatment, they will likely slowly worsen over time.

Many persons worry about the development of a syrinx unless they have an operation. Although in the past it was difficult to diagnose the presence of syrinx, today an MRI scan is a rapid and effective way to determine if one is present. Thus, worrying about the possibility that a syrinx will develop over time should not be a reason to choose surgery. A syrinx usually develops slowly and a follow-up MRI yearly can be done to determine if one is developing. Although no long-term studies are available to tell us what the Chiari I malformation does over time, most centers today have patients who have been found to have crowding from the Chiari I malformation but have minimal if any symptoms.

Syringomyelia

The best treatment for syringomyelia is to remove the block to normal spinal fluid flow. In patients with syringomyelia due to the Chiari I malformation, the goal is to create more room at the area of the foramen magnum (through a posterior fossa decompression as described above) and improve spinal fluid flow through the area. This will often result in the syrinx slowly decreasing in size, although it may not disappear completely (Figure 4). The important point is to keep the syrinx from growing and allow it to relax.

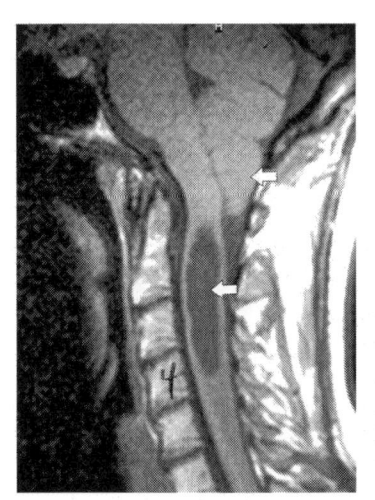

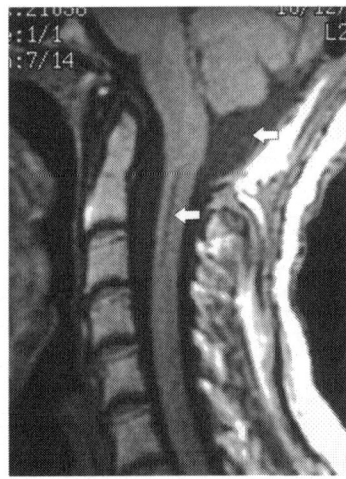

Figure 4: Pre and post-operative MRI scans of a person with the Chiari I Malformation and syringomyelia. Note the almost complete resolution of the syrinx in this case.

When syringomyelia is due to spinal trauma, release of the scar bands around the spinal cord can result in decrease in the size of the syrinx. When it is due to a spinal cord tumor, the best treatment is usually removal of the tumor if possible. When the cause of the syrinx is not known, the treatment decisions are more difficult. If the syrinx is small and the symptoms are under control, observation and follow-up MRI scans are appropriate. If the syrinx is enlarging or the symptoms are worsening, studies can be done looking for a tethered spinal cord, or rarely, the presence of a band within the spinal canal that is not visible on MRI scan. A myelogram study (injecting contrast material into the spinal canal) may be needed. When the cause is not found or the syrinx has not responded to other treatments, a shunt tube can be placed in the syrinx cavity. While some respond well to this treatment, concerns are that the catheter can become blocked and follow-up surgeries may be needed.

CHAPTER 9

SPECIAL CONSIDERATIONS IN CHIARI MALFORMATION

Children

The diagnosis of the Chiari I malformation is more difficult to make in young children and infants since they are unable to describe their symptoms. Before discussing the Chiari I malformation in children, it is important to review the Chiari II malformation.

All infants born with a myelomeningocele (a sac of tissue on the back of the spine, usually in the lower back) have the Chiari II malformation. Often, myelomeningocele is diagnosed in utero by ultrasound, thus allowing for a plan of care to be formulated prior to birth. Most of these infants require surgical repair of the myelomeningocele shortly after birth. Children with Chiari II carry a higher morbidity and mortality than children with Chiari I. The classic symptoms of Chiari II malformation in infants includes breathing difficulty, failure to gain weight or weight loss due to inadequate feeding capabilities, frequent vomiting, choking or difficulty swallowing, inability to cry normally, and apnea (occasionally stops breathing for short periods of time). Infants can rapidly progress in symptoms to life-threatening neurologic and respiratory emergency, requiring immediate treatment. An infant with respiratory stridor (difficult noisy breathing) should be evaluated in an emergency room immediately, as this can rapidly lead to apnea (cessation of breathing).

The Chiari I malformation also occurs in infants, but is uncommon. Infants may be inconsolable due to pain. Older infants may have difficulty swallowing, or frequent choking, and may be thought to have failure to thrive syndrome. Toddlers with the Chiari I malformation may hold their head and cry or scream out in pain, signifying headaches. Children with severe compression of the lower cranial nerve can have vocal cord dysfunction. Some children will vomit frequently for no apparent reason. Cases have been reported of children who have episodes of anger or rage due to unexpressed pain. Older toddlers may have balance problems and tend to fall frequently. Some young children will hold their head while straining (such as during a bowel movement) in attempt to suppress the head pain. A child may avoid bending over to pick up an object from the floor due to increased head pain during this activity. Some children will restrict their normal play activities or laughter due to unexpressed pain.

Older children often display disorders of the cerebellum by gait ataxia, stumbling, or falling. Increasing clumsiness in running can signify compression of the upper cervical spinal area. Weakness of the arms and hands can also be noted as changes in penmanship, inability to perform fine motor skills (such as tying shoes, buttoning buttons, or brushing the teeth). The child who could once throw a softball or run during recess may become unable to coordinate his/her movements. Neck pain may manifest by the child holding their neck or avoiding activities that require neck movement.

Adolescents

Adolescents more commonly have Chiari type I malformation unless they were previously diagnosed with myelomeningocele as an infant, or they have evidence of spina bifida occulta. Adolescents are often able to express and describe their symptoms more clearly than children. Most often, these young patients will describe symptoms that worsen with athletic activities, such as running, sports, and cheerleading. Many will report onset of symptoms after an injury in sports, such as football or softball. Some teenagers will limit their social activities due to pain and fatigue. Adolescents may also have a slightly higher occurrence of syncopal episodes (passing out or fainting). Memory and concentration difficulties may affect the teenager's ability to maintain their academic requirements. Teenagers who at one time participated in extracurricular activities may avoid such behavior due to pain or fatigue.

Compression of the lower cranial nerves or cerebellum can lead to symptoms such as dysphagia (swallowing difficulties), nausea, ataxia (balance problems) or upper extremity weakness. Changes in fine motor tasks of the hands can be noted in penmanship and personal care skills. Memory and cognitive difficulty can lead to decline in academic performance. Some teenagers will report neck, back, or extremity pain or numbness. The majority of symptoms reported in the adolescent age group are similar to those of the adults with Chiari I malformation.

Elderly

Some elderly persons will have symptoms that have been present "all their life," while others will have a new onset of symptoms attributable to the Chiari I malformation over the age of 60 years. It is difficult to understand why the symptoms begin so much later in life in some persons. Many elderly patients will report increased swallowing difficulty or gait imbalance as the primary symptom. Vertigo and dizziness are among the more common complaints for which the elderly person may seek medical attention. Although these symptoms can be attributable to multiple other causes in an elderly person, the radiographic evidence of Chiari I malformation should be considered a possible contributing factor. Treatment options remain the same for patients over the age of 60 years, however concurrent medical illnesses may pose a higher surgical risk. Age alone should not be a determining factor in the decision to proceed with surgery, or to avoid surgery for a person over age 60. Many persons over age 60 recover well after surgical decompression, and report an improvement in their post-surgical quality of life. The individual's specific risks and benefits should be carefully considered when developing a plan of care for the elderly population.

Pregnancy

Many women with the Chiari I malformation have normal pregnancies without symptoms. In fact, most of the women who are diagnosed with radiographic evidence of Chiari I malformation over the age of 40 years have likely already had children with no specific complications related to Chiari. The specific risks of each individual should be considered when counseling women on pregnancy in relation to Chiari malformation. The Chiari I malformation does seem to run in some families, but probably not more than in 12% of families with an affected member. In-utero birth defects, such as myelomeningocele can be determined by ultrasound prior to delivery of a baby.

There is very little in the English literature regarding the risks of pregnancy in the presence of Chiari I malformation. The main risk of epidural anesthesia is the possibility of puncture of the dura. This may result in post-lumbar puncture headache, which is often treated with a blood patch. However, a more troubling complication may be a spinal fluid leak, resulting in further descent of the cerebellar tonsils. This may cause worsening symptoms, and the possibility of further compression of the posterior fossa. The risk of general anesthesia in the case of a caesarean section may include hyperextension of the neck, resulting in increased symptoms. There is also a risk of increased intracranial pressure during general anesthesia. The exact risks of increased intracranial pressure from general anesthesia are uncertain. However, a recent series by Mueller & Oro' (see references), of seven women with Chiari I malformation with and without syringomyelia, both before and after surgical decompression revealed no specific contraindication to pregnancy, and no specific complication from either vaginal birth or caesarean section. It is best for the pregnant woman, or a woman who is planning a pregnancy to fully discuss all current symptoms, treatments, surgeries and any complications with their obstetrician prior to delivery to determine the specific risks for the individual.

CHAPTER 10

SUMMARY

This book reviews a disorder of the posterior structures of the skull and brain believed to occur during prenatal development. Some people may never experience significant symptoms related to the Chiari malformation, while others may develop worsening symptoms that eventually affect their quality of life. Modern diagnosis and treatment have been useful in helping many individuals suffering from this disorder resume a productive life with few and sometimes no symptoms, while some persons remain affected despite extensive treatment. That is the challenge before us.

Future progress in the diagnosis and management of the Chiari malformations will depend on several factors. A better understanding of the cause, the incidence within the population, and the natural history will provide persons with the disorder and their families, as well as health care providers, a more solid foundation on which to make decisions. People who suffer for years prior to diagnosis often do not respond as well to medical or surgical treatment, thus earlier recognition of the Chiari malformation can lead to treatment before personal or professional life becomes disrupted. While the MRI has dramatically improved the ability to diagnose neurological disorders including CM, further advancements are needed to help better visualize and measure the effects on neurological tissues. Improved studies on cerebrospinal fluid physiology should allow more precise measurements of the impact on spinal fluid flow and should clarify the mechanism of syrinx formation.

Working with the primary care provider, neurologist, neurosurgeon, and other specialists will remain important in sorting out which of the many possible causes are responsible for the symptoms experienced. Improvements in medical management and surgical care should enhance the effectiveness of treatment for those affected. The modern lifestyle with its potential lack of physical activity and sometimes, marginal nutrition, may also play a role in aggravating symptoms and hindering full recovery. The importance of diet, sleep and physical activity in neurological health are increasingly being recognized.

Of everything a person with the Chiari I malformation can do, the most important is to participate in their own health care. That is the spirit of this book. The more one knows, the better the chances are for one to return to a healthy life. The authors hope we have shed some light on this disorder. We welcome any suggestions for improvement of future editions.

Chiari & Syringomyelia Articles

Aboulezz AO, Sartor K, Geyer CA, Gado MH (1985). Position of Cerebellar tonsils in the normal population and in patients with Chiari Malformation: a quantative approach with MR imaging. Journal of Computer Assisted Tomography, 9(6), 1033-1036.

Achiron A, Kuritzky A. (1990). Dysphagia as the sole manifestation of adult type I Arnold-Chiari malformation. Neurology, 40, 186-187.

Aldern TD, Ojemann JG, Park TS (2001). Surgical treatment of Chiari I malformation: indications and approaches. Neurosurgery Focus, 11(1), 1-5.

Ali MM, Russell N, Awada A, McLean D (1996). A craniocervical malformation presenting as acute respiratory failure. The Journal of Emergency Medicine, 14(5), 569-572.

Allsopp GM, Karkanevatos A, Bickerton RC (2000). Abductor vocal fold palsy as a manifestation of type one Arnold Chiari malformation. Journal of Laryngology & Otology, 114(3): 221-3.

Alperin N, Kulkarni K, Roitberg B, Loth F, Pandian NK, Mafee, MF, Foroohar M, Lichtor T (2001). Analysis of magnetic resonance imaging-based blood and cerebrospinal fluid flow measurements in patients with Chiari I malformation: a system approach. Neurosurgical Focus, 11(1), 1-10.

Alvarez D, Requena I, Arias M, Valdes L, Pereiro I, De la Torre R (1995). Acute respiratory failure as the first sign of Arnold-Chiari malformation associated with syringomyelia. European Respiratory Journal, 8, 661-663.

Alzate JC, Kothbauer KF, Jallo GI, Epstein FJ (2001). Treatment of Chiari type I malformation in patients with and without syringomyelia: a consecutive series of 66 cases. Neurosurgical Focus, 11 (1) 1-9.

Amir TA, El-Shamam OM (1997) Chiari malformation type I: a new MRI classification. Magnetic Resonance Imaging 15 (4), 397-403.

Anderson RC, Dowling KC, Feldstein NA, Emerson RG (2003). Chiari I malformation: potential role for intraoperative electrophysiologic monitoring. Journal of Clinical Neurophysiology, 20(1), 65-72.

Anderson RC, Emerson RG, Dowling KC, Feldstein, NA (2003). Improvement in brainstem auditory evoked potentials after suboccipital decompression in patients with Chiari I malformations. Journal of Neurosurgery, 98, 459-464.

Arai S, Ohtsuka Y, Moriya H, Kitahara H, Minami S (1993). Scoliosis associated with syringomyelia. Spine, 18(12), 1591-1592.

Armonda RA, Citrin CM, Foley KT, Ellenbogen RG (1994). Quantitative Cine-mode magnetic resonance imaging of Chiari I malformations: an analysis of cerebrospinal fluid dynamics. Neurosurgery, 35(2), 214-224.

Arnett B (2003). Arnold-Chiari malformation (History of Neurology). Archives of Neurology, 60(6), 898-900.

Arora P, Behari S, Banerji D, Chhabra DK, Jain VK (2004). Factors influencing the outcome in symptomatic Chiari I malformation. Neurology India, 52(4):470-4.

Ball WS, Crone KR (1995). Chiari I Malformation: from Dr. Chiari to MR Imaging. Radiology, 195, 602-604.

Banerji NK, Millar HD (1974). Chiari malformation presenting in adult life. Brain, 97, 157-168.

Batzdorf U (2000). Primary spinal syringomyelia: a personal perspective. Neurosurgery Focus 8(3), 1-4.

Bauer A, Mueller DM, Oro JJ (2005). Arachnoid cyst resulting in tonsillar herniation and syringomyelia in a patient with achondroplasia: a case report. Neurosurgical Focus. Nov 15;19(5):E14.

Bejjani GK (2001). Definition of the adult Chiari malformation: a brief historical overview. Neurosurgical Focus, 11(1), 1-8.

Beuls EA, Vandersteen MA, Vanormelingen LM, Adriaensens PJ, Freling G, Herpers MJ, Gelan JM (1996). Deformation of the cervicomedullary junction and spinal cord in a surgically treated adult Chiari I hindbrain hernia associated with syringomyelia: a magnetic resonance microscopic and neuropathological study. Journal of Neurosurgery, 85, 701-708.

Bell WO, Charney EB, Bruce DA, Sutton LN, Schut L (1987). Symptomatic Arnold-Chiari malformation: review of experience with 22 cases. Journal of Neurosurgery, 66, 812-816.

Bindal AK, Dunsker SB, Tew JM (1995). Chiari I Malformation: Classification and management. Neurosurgery, 37(6): 1069-1074.

Black, P (2000). Cerebrospinal fluid leaks following spinal or posterior fossa surgery: use of fat grafts for prevention and repair. Neurosurgical Focus, 9(1), 1-4.

Blevins NH, Deschler DG, Kingdom TT, Lee KC (1997). Chiari I malformation presenting as vocal cord paralysis in the adult. Otolaryngology- Head & Neck Surgery, 117(6): S191-4.

Bloch S, Van Rensburg MJ, Danziger J (1974). The Arnold-Chiari malformation. Clinical Radiology, 25, 335-341.

Bogdanov EL, Heiss JD, Mendelevick EG, Mikhaylov IM, Haass A (2004). Clinical and neuroimaging features of "idiopathic" syringomyelia. Neurology, 62(5): 791-4.

Botelho RV, Bittencort LR, Rotta JM, Tufik S (2003). A Prospective controlled study of sleep respiratory events in patients with craniovertebral junction malformation. Journal of Neurosurgery, 99(6); 1004-9

Brugieres P, Idy-Peretti I, Iffenecker C, Parker F, Jolivet O, Hurth M, Gaston A, & Bittoun J (2000). CSF flow measurement in syringomyelia. American Journal of Neuroradiology, 21, 1785-1792.

Byard RW (1996). Mechanisms of sudden death and autopsy findings in patients with Arnold-Chiari malformation and ventriculoatrial catheters. American Journal of Forensic Medicine and Pathology, 17(3): 260-3.

Carmel PW, Markesbery WR (1972). Early descriptions of the Arnold-Chiari malformation. Journal of Neurosurgery, 37, 543-547.

Cavander RK, Schmidt JH (1995). Tonsillar ectopia and Chiari malformations: monozygotic triplets. Journal of Neurosurgery, 82, 497-500.

Chait GE, Barber HO (1979). Arnold-Chiari malformation: some otoneurological features. Journal of Otolaryngology, 8, 65-70.

Chang HS, Nakagawa H (2003). Hypothesis on the pathophysiology of syringomyelia based on simulation of cerebrospinal fluid dynamics. Journal of Neurology, Neurosurgery and Psychiatry, 74(3), 344-347.

Chantigian RC, Koehn MA, Ramin KD, Warner MA (2002). Chiari I malformation in parturients. Journal of Clinical Anesthesia, 14, 201-205.

Coria F, Quintana F, Rebollo, M, Combarros, O., Berciano, J. (1983). Occipital dysplasia and Chiari type I deformity in a family. Journal of the Neurological Sciences, 62, 147-158.

Corbett JJ, Butler AB, & Kaufman B (1976). Sneeze syncope, basilar invagination and Arnold-Chiari type I malformation. Journal of Neurology, Neurosurgery, and Psychiatry, 39, 381-384.

Couldwell WT, Zhang W, Allen R, Arce S, Stillerman CB (1998). Cerebellar contusion associated with Type I Chiari malformation following supratentorial head trauma: case report. Neurological Research, 20(1): 93-6.

Curnes JT, Oakes WJ, Boyko OB (1989). MR imaging of hindbrain deformity in Chiari II patients with and without symptoms of brainstem compression. American Journal of Neuroradiolgy,10(2): 293-302.

DelBigio MR, Deck JHN, MacDonald J.K (1992). Syrinx extending from conus medullaris to basal ganglia: a clinical, radiological, and pathological correlation. The Canadian Journal of Neurological Sciences, 20, 240-246.

Depreitere B, Van Calenberg, F, van Loon J, Goffin J. Plets C (2000). Posterior fossa decompression in syringomyelia associated with Chiari malformation: a retrospective analysis of 22 patients. Clinical Neurology and Neurosurgery, 102, 91-96.

Dobkin BH (1977). The adult Chiari malformation. Bulletin of the Los Angeles Neurological Societies, 42(1), 23-7.

Dyste GN, Menezes AH, VanGilder JC (1989). Symptomatic Chiari Malformations: an analysis of presentation, management, and long-term outcome. Journal of Neurosurgery, 71, 159-168.

Ellenbogen RG, Armonda RA, Shaw DWW, Winn HR (2000). Toward a rational treatment of Chiari I malformation and syringomyelia. Neurosurgical Focus, 8(3), 1-10.

Elster AD, Chen, YM (1992). Chiari I Malformations: clinical and radiologic reappraisal. Radiology, 183(2), 347-353

Elta GH, Caldwell CA, Nostrant TT (1996). Esophageal dysphagia as the sole symptom in Type I Chiari malformation. Digestive Diseases and Sciences, 41(3), 512-515.

Emery E, Redondo A, Rey A (1997). Syringomyelia and Arnold-Chiari in scoliosis initially classified as idiopathic: experience with 25 patients. European Spine Journal, 6, 158-162.

Enzmann DR, Pelc NJ (1992). Brain motion: measurement with phase-contrast MR imaging. Radiology, 185, 653-660.

Enzmann DR, Pelc NJ (1993). Cerebrospinal fluid flow measured by phase-contrast cine MR. American Journal of Neuroradiology, 14, 1301-1306.

Erkan K, Unal F, Kiris T, Karalar T (2000). Treatment of terminal syringomyelia in association with tethered cord syndrome: clinical outcomes with and without syrinx drainage. Neurosurgical Focus, 8(3), 1-6.

Faria MA, Spector RH, Tindall GT (1980). Downbeat nystagmus as the salient manifestation of the Arnold-Chiari malformation. Surgical Neurology, 13, 333-336.

Fischbein NJ, Dillon, WP, Cobbs C, Weinstein PR (1999). The presyrinx state: a reversible myelopathic condition that may precede syringomyelia. American Journal of Neuroradiology, 20, 7-20.

Fuller R, Stanners A (2000). A cough, then respiratory failure. The Lancet, 356.

Garland EM, Robertson D (2001). Chiari I Malformation as a cause of orthostatic intolerance symptoms: a media myth? The American Journal of Medicine, 546-552.

Gentry JB, Gonzalez JM, Blacklock JB (2001). Respiratory failure caused by Chiari I Malformation with associated syringomyelia. Clinical Neurology and Neurosurgery, 103, 43-45.

Gezen F, Kahraman S, Ziyal IM, Canakci Z, Bakir A (2000). Application of syringosubarachnoid shunt through key-hole laminectomy. Neurosurgery Focus, 8(3), 1-3.

Ghanem I B, Londono C, Delalande O, Dubousset JF (1997). Chiari I malformation associated with syringomyelia and scoliosis. Spine, 22(12), 1313-1317.

Gillespie JE, Jenkins JPR, Metcalfe RA, Isherwood I (1986). Magnetic resonance imaging in syringomyelia. Acta Radiologica-Supplementum, 239-241.

Goel A, Desai K (2000). Surgery for syringomyelia: an analysis based on 163 surgical cases. Acta Neurochirurgica, 142(3): 293-301.

Greenlee JW, Donovan KA, Hasan DM, Menezes AH (2002). Chiari I malformation in the very young child: the spectrum of presentations and experience in 31 children under age 6 years. Pediatrics, 110(6), 1212-1219.

Greitz, D, Wirestam R, Franck A, Nordell B, Thomsen C, Stahlberg F (1992). Pulsatile brain movement and associated hydrodynamics studied by magnetic resonance phase imaging. Neuroradiology, 34, 370-380.

Guyotat J, Bret P, Jouanneau E, Ricci AC, Lapras C (1998). Syringomyelia associated with type I Chiari malformation. A 21-year retrospective study on 75 cases treated by foramen magnum decompression with a special emphasis on the value of tonsils resection Acta Neurochir (Wien), 140, 745-754.

Hampton F, Williams B, & Loizou LA (1982). Syncope as a presenting feature of hindbrain herniation with syringomyelia. Journal of Neurology, Neurosurgery and Psychiatry, 45, 919-922.

Haroun RI, Guarnieri M, Meadow JJ, Kraut M, Carson BS (2000). Current opinions for the treatment of syringomyelia and chiari malformations: survey of the Pediatric Section of the American Association of Neurological Surgeons. Pediatric Neurosurgery, 33(6): 11-7.

Haughton VM, Korosec FR, Medow JE, Dolar MT, Iskandar BJ (2003). Peak systolic and diastolic CSF velocity in the foramen magnum in adult patients with Chiari I malformations and in normal control participants. American Journal of Neuroradiology, 24, 169-176.

Heiss JD, Patronas N, DeVroom HL, Shawker T, Ennis R, Kammerer W, Eidsath A, Talbot T, Morris J, Eskioglu E, Oldfield EH (1999). Elucidating the pathophysiology of syringomyelia. Journal of Neurosurgery, 91, 553-562.

Herman MD, Cheek WR, Storrs BB (1990). Two siblings with the Chiari I malformation. Pediatric Neurosurgery, 16, 183-184.

Hida K, Iwasaki Y, Koyanagi I, Sawamura Y, Abe, H (1995). Surgical indications and results of foramen magnum decompression versus syringosubarachnoid shunting for syringomyelia associated with Chiari I malformation. Neurosurgery 37(4), 673-678.

Hilton EL, Henderson LJ (2003). Neurosurgical considerations in posttraumatic syringomyelia. Journal of the Association of Perioperative Registered Nurses, 77(1), 135-156.

Holly LT, Batzdorf U (2002). Slitlike syrinx cavities: a persistent central canal. Journal of Neurosurgery: Spine 2, 97, 161-165.

Holly LT, Johnson JP, Masciopinto JE, Batzdorf U (2000). Treatment of posttraumatic syringomyelia with extradural decompressive surgery. Neurosurgical Focus, 8(3), 1-6.

Huang PP, Constantini S (1994). Acquired Chiari I malformation. Case report. Journal of Neurosurgery, 80(6): 1099-102.

Hudgins RJ (1999). Paroxysmal rage as a presenting symptoms of the Chiari I malformation. Journal of Neurosurgery, 91, 328-329.

Inoue Y, Nemoto Y, Ohata K, Daikokuya H, Tashiro T, Shakudo M, Nagai K, Nakayama K, Yamada R (2001). Syringomyelia associated with adhesive spinal arachnoiditis: MRI. Neuroradiology, 43, 325-330.

Ireland PD, Mickelsen D, Rodenhouse TG, Bakos RS, Goldstein B (1996). Evaluation of the autonomic cardiovascular response in Arnold-Chiari deformities and cough syncope syndrome. Archives of Neurology, 53, 526-531.

Iskandar BJ, Hedlund GL, Grabb PA, Oakes WJ (2000). The resolution of syringohydromyelia without hindbrain herniation after posterior fossa decompression. Neurosurgical Focus (8) 1-5.

Isu T, Sasaki H, Takamura H, Kobayashi N. (1993). Foramen magnum decompression with removal of the outer layer of the dura as treatment for syringomyelia occurring with Chiari I malformation. Neurosurgery, 33(5), 845-850.

Iwasaki Y, Hida K, Koyanagi I, Abe H (2000). Reevaluation of syringosubarachnoid shunt for syringomyelia with Chiari malformation. Neurosurgery, 46(2): 407-12.

Jacome DE (2001). Blepharoclonus and Arnold-Chiari malformation. Acta Neurologica Scandinavica, 104(2), 113-117.

Kahn T, Muller E, Lewin JS, Modder U (1992). MR measurement of spinal CSF flow with the RACE technique. Journal of Computer Assisted Tomography, 16(1), 54-61.

Khurana RK (1991). Headache spectrum in Arnold-Chiari malformation. Headache, 31, 151-155.

Klekamp J, Iaconetta G, Giorgio MD, Samii M. (2001). Spontaneous resolution of Chiari I Malformation and syringomyelia: case report and review of the literature. Neurosurgery, 48(3), 664-667.

Koch CA, Heiss JD, Pacak K, Krakoff J, Winer KK, Wassermann EM (2000). Chiari malformation type 1 and osteoporosis. Neurosurgery Review, 23: 171-2.

Kokmen E, Marsh WR, Baker HL (1985). Magnetic resonance imaging in syringomyelia. Neurosurgery, 17(2), 267-270.

Lacy BE, Zayat E, Crowell MD (2001). Generalized intestinal dysmotility in a patient with syringomyelia. American Journal of Gastroenterology, 96(4): 1282-5.

Leong WK, Kermode AG (2001). Acute deterioration in Chiari type I malformation after chiropractic cervical manipulation. Journal of Neurology, Neurosurgery and Psychiatry, 70, 816-817.

Lesoin F, Petit H, Thomas CE, Viaud C, Baleriaux D, Jomin M (1986). Use of the syringoperitoneal shunt in the treatment of syringomyelia. Surgical Neurology, 25, 131-136.

Levy LM (2003). MR identification of Chiari pathophysiology by using spatial and temporal CSF flow indices and implications for syringomyelia. American Journal of Neuroradiology, 24, 165-66.

Levy LM, DiChiro G (1990). MR phase imaging and cerebrospinal fluid flow in the head and spine. Neuroradiology, 32, 399-406.

Levy WJ, Mason L, Hahn JF (1983). Chiari malformation presenting in adults: a surgical experience in 127 cases. Neurosurgery, 12(4). 377-390.

Li KC, & Chui MC (1987). Conventional and CT metrizamide myelography in Arnold-Chiari I malformation and syringomyelia. American Journal of Neuroradiology, 8, 11-17.

Mampalam TJ, Andrews BT, Gelb D, Ferriero D, Pitts LH (1988). Presentation of type I Chiari malformation after head trauma. Neurosurgery, 23(6); 760-2.

Mariani C, Cislaghi MG, Barbieri S, Filizzolo F, DiPalma F, Farina E, D'Alberti G, Scarlato G (1991). The natural history and results of surgery in 50 cases of syringomyelia, Journal of Neurology, 238, 433-438.

Matsumoto T, Symon L (1989). Surgical management of syringomyelia-current results. Surgical Neurology, 32, 258-265.

McComb JG (1993). The usefulness of phase-contrast MR measurement of cerebrospinal fluid flow. American Journal of Neuroradiology, 14, 1309-1310.

Meadows J, Kraut M, Guarnieri M, Haroun RI, Carson BJ (2000). Asymptomatic Chiari type I malformations identified on magnetic resonance imaging. Journal of Neurosurgery, 92, 920-926.

Menick BJ (2001). Phase-contrast magnetic resonance imaging of cerebrospinal fluid flow in the evaluation of patients with Chiari I malformation. Neurosurgical Focus, 11(1), 1-4.

Meves SH, Postert T, Przuntek H, Buttner, T (2000). Acute brainstem symptoms associated with syringomyelia. European Neurology, 43, 47-49.

Mikulis DJ, Diaz O, Egglin TK, Sanchez R (1992). Variance of the position of the cerebellar tonsils with age: preliminary report. Radiology, 183, 725-728.

Milhorat TH (2000). Classification of syringomyelia. Neurosurgical Focus, 8(3), 1-6.

Milhorat TH, Chou MW, Trinidad EM, Kula RW, Mandell M, Wolpert C, Speer MC (1999). Chiari I Malformation redefined: clinical and radiographic findings for 364 symptomatic patients. Neurosurgery, 44(5), 1005-1017.

Milhorat TH, Johnson WD, Miller JI, Bergland RM, Hollenberg-Sher J (1992). Surgical treatment of syringomyelia based on magnetic resonance imaging criteria. Neurosurgery, 31(2), 231-245.

Mobbs R, Teo C (2001). Endoscopic assisted posterior fossa decompression. Journal of Clinical Neuroscience, 8(4), 343-344.

Mohr PD, Strang FA, Sambrook MA, & Boddie HG (1977). The clinical and surgical features in 40 patients with primary cerebellar ectopia (adult Chiari Malformation). Quarterly Journal of Medicine, 181, 85-96

Mueller, D. (2001). Brainstem conundrum: the Chiari I malformation. Journal of the American Academy of Nurse Practitioners, 13(4), 154-159.

Mueller DM, Oro' JJ (2004). Prospective analysis of presenting symptoms among 265 patients with radiographic evidence of Chiari malformation type I with or without syringomyelia. Journal of the American Academy of Nurse Practitioners,16(3): 134-138.

Mueller DM, Oro' JJ (2005). Prospective analysis of self-perceived quality of life before and after posterior fossa decompression in 112 patients with or without syringomyelia. Neurosurgical Focus, 18(2), 1-6.

Munshi I, Frim D, Stine-Reyes R, Weir BK, Hekmatpanah J, Brown F (2000). Effects of posterior fossa decompression with and without duraplasty on Chiari malformation associated hydromyelia. Neurosurgery, 46(6): 1384-9.

Murayama K, Mamiya K, Nozaki K, Sakurai K, Sengoku K, Osamu T, Iwasaki H (2001). Cesarean section in a patient with syringomyelia. Canadial Journal of Anesthesia, 48, 474-477.

Narotam PK, vanDellen JR, Bhoola KD (1995). A clinicopathological study of collagen sponge as a dural graft in neurosurgery. Journal of Neurosurgery, 82, 406-412.

Nash J, Cheng JS, Meyer GA, Remler BF (2002). Chiari type I malformation: overview of diagnosis and treatment. Wisconsin Medical Journal 101(8), 35-40.

Nathadwarawala KM, Richards CA, Lawrie B, Thomas GO, Wiles CM(1992). Recurrent aspiration due to Arnold-Chiari type I malformation. British Medical Journal, 304, 565-566.

Nishikawa M, Sakamoto H, Hakuba A, Nakinishi N, Inoue Y (1997). Pathogenesis of Chiari malformation: a morphometric study of the posterior cranial fossa. Journal of Neurosurgery, 86, 40-47.

Nishizawa S, Yokoyama T, Yokota N, Tokuyama T, Ohata S (2001). Incidentally identified syringomyelia associated with Chiari I malformations: is early interventional surgery necessary? Neurosurgery, 49(3), 637-641.

Njemanze PC, Beck OJ (1989). MR- Gated intracranial CSF dynamics: evaluation of CSF pulsatile flow. American Journal of Neuroradiology, 10, 77-80.

Ohara S, Nagai H, Matsumoto T, Banno T (1988). MR imaging of CSF pulsatory flow and its relation to intracranial pressure. Journal of Neurosurgery, 69, 675-682.

Oldfield EH, Kuraszko K, Shawker TH, Patronas NJ (1994). Pathophysiology of syringomyelia associated with Chiari I malformation of the cerebellar tonsils. Journal of Neurosurgery, 80, 3-15.

Olivero WC, Dinh DH (1992). Chiari I malformation with traumatic syringomyelia and spontaneous resolution: case report and literature review. Neurosurgery, 30(5), 758-760.

Omer S, al-Kawi MZ, Bohlega S, Bouchama A, Mclean D (1996). Respiratory arrest: a complication of Arnold chiari malformation in adults. European Neurology, 36(1): 36-8

Ono A, Ueyama K, Okada A, Echigoya N, Yokoyama T, Harata S (2002). Adult scoliosis in syringomyelia associated with Chiari I malformation. Spine, 2002; 27(2) E23-8

O'Reilly SA., Toffol GJ (1995). Adult Arnold-Chiari malformation: a postpartum case presentation. Journal of the American Osteopathic Association, 95(10), 607-609.

Pamir MN, Ozer AF, Zihr TA, Gurmen N, Erzen C (1991). CT myelography in communicating syringomyelia. European Journal of Radiology, 12, 47-52.

Padney A, Robinson S, Cohen AR (2001). Cerebellar fits in children with Chiari I malformation. Neurosurgical Focus, 11(1), 1-4.

Palma V, Sinisi L, Andreone V, Fazio N, Serra LL, Ambrosio G, De Michele G (1993). Hindbrain hernia headache and syncope in type I Arnold-Chiari malformation. Acta Neurologica,15(6): 457-61.

Pare LS, Batzdorf U (1998). Syringomyelia persistence after Chiari decompression as a result of pseudomeningocele formation: implications for syrinx pathogenesis: report of three cases. Neurosurgery, 43(4), 945-948.

Parker JD, Broberg JC, Napolitano PG (2002). Maternal Arnold-Chiari type I malformation and syringomyelia: a labor management dilemma. American Journal of Perinatology, 19(4), 445-450.

Parker EC, Teo C, Rahman S, Brodsky MC (2000). Complete resolution of hypertension after decompression of Chiari I malformation. Skull Base Surgery, 10(3), 149-152.

Pascual J, Oterino A, & Berciano J (1992). Headache in type I Chiari malformation. Neurology, 42, 1591-1521.

Pasupuleti DV, Vedre A (2005). Postural orthostatic tachycardia warrants investigation of Chiari I malformation as a possible cause. Cardiology, 103(1):55-6.

Paul KS, Lye RH, Strang FA, & Dutton J (1983). Arnold-Chiari malformation: review of 71 cases. Journal of Neurosurgery, 58, 183-187.

Pidcock FS, Sandel ME, Faro S (1994). Late onset of syringomyelia after traumatic brain injury: association with Chiari I malformation. Archives of Physical Medicine and Rehabilitation, 75(6) 695-8.

Pillay PK, Awad IA, Little JR, Hahn JF (1991). Symptomatic Chiari malformation in adults: a new classification based on magnetic resonance imaging with clinical and prognostic significance. Neurosurgery, 28(5), 639-645.

Pinna G, Alessandrini F, Alfieri A, Rossi M, & Bricolo A (2000). Cerebrospinal fluid flow dynamics study in Chiari I malformation: implications for syrinx formation. Neurosurgical Focus, 8(3), 1-8.

Pollack IF, Pang D, Kocoshis S, Putnam P (1992). Neurogenic dysphagia resulting from Chiari malformations. Neurosurgery, 30, 709-719.

Pringle RG (2000). Post-traumatic syringomyelia. Spinal Cord, 2000; 38(3): 199.

Quencer RM, Donovan Post MJ, Hinks RS (1990). Cine MR in the evaluation of normal and abnormal CSF flow: intracranial and intraspinal studies. Neuroradiology, 32, 371-391.

Quigley MF, Iskandar B, Quigley MA, Nicosia M, Haughton V (2004). Cerebrospinal fluid flow in foramen magnum: Temporal and spatial patterns at MR imaging in volunteers and in patients with Chiari I malformation. Radiology, 232: 229-236.

Rao VRK, Joseph S, Mandalam KR, Jain SK, Gupta AK, Unni NR, Rao AS, Mohan PK (1991). Syringohydromyelia: radiological evaluation of 82 patients in a developing country. Clinical Radiology, 44, 165-171.

Rekate HL, Nadkarni TD, Teaford PA, Wallace D (1999). Brainstem dysfunction in Chiari malformation presenting as profound hypoglycemia: presentation of four cases, review of the literature and conjecture as to mechanism. Neurosurgery, 45(2), 386-391.

Rodolico C, Girlanda P, Nicolosi C, Vita G, Bonsignore M, Tortorella G (2003). Chiari I malformation mimicking myasthenia gravis. Journal of Neurology, Neurosurgery and Psychiatry, 74(3), 393.

Rosetti P, Taib NOB, Brotchi J, De Witte O (1999). Arnold Chiari type I malformation presenting as a trigeminal neuralgia: case report. Neurosurgery, 44(5), 1122-1124.

Royo-Salvador MB, Sole'-Llenas J, Domenech JM, Gonzalea-Adrio R (2005). Results of the section of the filum terminale in 20 patients with syringomyelia and Chiari malformation. Acta Neurochurgica, 515-523.

Rudick RA, Schiffer RB, Schwetz K, Herndon RM (1986). Multiple Sclerosis: the problem of incorrect diagnosis. Archives of Neurology, 43, 578-583.

Runge VM, Gelblum DY, Wood ML (1990). 3-D imaging of the CNS. Neuroradiology, 32, 356-366.

Samii C, Mobius E, Weber W, Heienbrok HW, Berlit P (1999). Pseudo Chiari type I malformation secondary to cerebrospinal fluid leakage. Journal of Neurology, 246, 162-164.

Sansur CA, Heiss JD, DeVroom HL, Eskioglu E, Ennis R, Oldfield EH (2003). Pathophysiology of headache associated with cough in patients with Chiari I malformation. Journal of Neurosurgery, 98, 453-458.

Schaan M, Jaksche H (2001). Comparison of different operative modalities in post-traumatic syringomyelia: preliminary report. European Spine Journal, 10, 135-140.

Schijman E, Steinbok P (2004). International survey on the management of Chiari I malformation and syringomyelia. Childs Nervous System, 20: 341-348.

Seijo-Martinez M, Castro del Rio, M, Conde C, Brasa J, Vila O (2004). Cluster-like headache: association with cervical syringomyelia and Arnold Chiari malformation. Cephalalgia, 24(2), 140-2.

Sellery GR (2001). Intraoperative problem during surgery for Chiari malformation. Canadian Journal of Anesthesia, 48, 718.

Semple DA, McClure JH (1996). Arnold-Chiari malformation in pregnancy. Anaesthesia, 51, 580-582.

Sheehan JM, Jane JA (2000). Resolution of tonsillar herniation and syringomyelia after supratentorial tumor resection: case report and review of the literature. Neurosurgery, 47(1), 233-235.

Silver JR (2001). History of post-traumatic syringomyelia: post traumatic syringomyelia prior to 1920. Spinal Cord, 39, 176-183.

Sindou M, Chavez-Machuca J, Hashish H (2002). Craniocervical decompression for Chiari type I malformation, adding extreme lateral foramen magnum opening and expansile duroplasty with arachnoid preservation. Technique and long-term functional results in 44 consecutive adult cases. Acta Neurochirurgica, 144(10); 1005-1019.

Speer MC, George TM, Enterline DS, Franklin A, Wolpert, CM, Milhorat TH (2000). A genetic hypothesis for Chiari I malformation with or without syringomyelia. Neurosurgical Focus, 8(3), 1-4.

Stevens JM, Serva WAD, Kendall BE, Valentine AR, Ponsford JR (1993). Chiari malformation in adults: relation of morphological aspects to clinical features and operative outcome. Journal of Neurology, Neurosurgery and Psychiatry, 56, 1072-1077.

Stevenson KL (2004). Chiari type II malformation: past, present, and future. Neurosurgical Focus, 16(2), 1-7.

Stovner LJ (1993). Headache associated with the Chiari type I malformation. Headache, 33, 175-181.

Stovner LJ (1992). Headache and Chiari type I malformation: occurrence in female monozygotic twins and first-degree relatives. Cephalalgia, 12, 304-307.

Stovner LJ, Cappelen J, Nilsen G, Sjaastad O (1992). The Chiari type I malformation in two monozygotic twins and first-degree relatives. Annals of Neurology, 31, 220-222.

Stovner LJ, Rinck P (1992). Syringomyelia in Chiari malformation: relation to extent of cerebellar tissue herniation. Neurosurgery, 31(5), 913-917.

Sun JC, Steinbok P, Cochrane DD (2000). Spontaneous resolution and recurrence of a Chiari I malformation and associated syringomyelia. Journal of Neurosurgery (Spine2), 92, 207-210.

Susman J, Jones C, Wheatley D (1989). Arnold-Chiari malformation: a diagnostic challenge. AFP, 39(3), 207-211.

Tashiro K, Fukazawa T, Moriwaka F, Hamada T, Isu T, Iwasaki Y, Abe H (1987). Syringomyelic syndrome: clinical features in 31 cases confirmed by CT myelography or magnetic resonance imaging. Journal of Neurology, 235, 26-30.

Takeuchi A, Miyamoto K, Sugiyama S, Saitou M, Hosoe, H, Shimizu K. (2003). Spinal arachnoid cysts associated with syringomyelia: report of two cases and a review of the literature. Journal of Spinal Disorders and Techniques, 16(2), 207-211.

Terae S, Miyasaka K, Abe S, Abe H, Tashiro K. (1994). Increased pulsatile movement of the hindbrain in syringomyelia associated with the Chiari malformation: cone-MRI with presaturation bolus tracking. Neuroradiology, 36, 125-129.

Todor DR, Mu HT, Milhorat TH (2000). Pain and syringomyelia: a review. Neurosurgical Focus, 8(3), 1-6.

Tominaga T, Koshu K, Ogawa A, Yoshimoto T. (1991). Transoral decompression evaluated by Cine-mode magnetic resonance imaging: a case of basilar impression accompanied by Chiari Malformation. Neurosurgery, 28(6), 883-885.

Tubbs RS, McGirt MJ, Oakes WJ (2003). Surgical experience in 130 pediatric patients with Chiari malformations. Journal of Neurosurgery, 99(2), 291-296.

Tubbs RS, Wellons JC III, Blount JP, & Oakes, WJ (2004). Syringomyelia in twin brothers discordant for Chiari I malformation: case report. Journal of Child Neurology, 19(6):459-62.

Tubbs RS, Wellons, JC, Oakes WJ (2002). Asymmetry of tonsillar ectopia in Chiari I malformation. Pediatric Neurosurgery, 37(4), 199-202.

Tubbs RS, Smyth MD, Wellons JC III, & Oakes WJ (2003). Hemihypertrophy and the Chiari I malformation. Pediatric Neurosurgery, 38(5): 258-261.

Tubbs RS, Wellons JC III, Smyth MD, Bartolucci AA, Grabb PA (2003). Children with growth hormone deficiency and Chiari I malformation: a morphometric analysis of the posterior cranial fossa. Pediatric Neurosurgery, 38(6): 324-8.

Tubbs RS, Elton S, Grabb P, Dockery SE, Bartolucci AA, Oakes WJ (2001). Analysis of the posterior fossa in children with the Chiari 0 malformation. Neurosurgery, 48(5), 1050-1054.

Iskandar BJ, Hedlund GL, Grabb PA, Oaks WJ (1998). The resolution of syringohydromyelia without hindbrain herniation after posterior fossa decompression. Journal of Neurosurgery, 212-216.

Vanaclocha V, Saiz-Sapena N (1997). Duraplasty with freeze-dried cadaveric dura versus occipital pericranium for Chiari type I Malformation: comparative study. Acta Neurochir (Wien), 139, 112-119.

Vanhatalo S, Paetau R, Mustonen K, Hernesniemi J, Riikonen R (2000). Posttraumatic tremor and Arnold Chiari malformation: no sign of compression, but cure after surgical decompression. Movement Disorders, 15(3): 581-3.

Ventureya ECG, Aziz HA, Vassilyadi M (2003). The role of cine flow MRI in children with Chiari I malformation. Child's Nervous System, 19(2): 109-113.

Vinas FC, Pilitsis J, Wilner H (2001). Spontaneous resolution of a syrinx. Journal of Clinical Neuroscience, 8(2), 170-172.

Weber PC, Cass SP (1993). Neurotologic manifestations of Chiari I malformation. Otolaryngology- Head and Neck Surgery, 109(5), 853-860.

Weig SG, Buckthal PE, Choi SK, Zellem RT (1991). Recurrent syncope as the presenting symptom of Arnold-Chiari malformation. Neurology, 41, 1673-1674.

Welch K, Shillito J, Strand R, Fischer EG, Winston KR (1981). Chiari I malformation- an acquired disorder? Journal of Neurosurgery, 55, 604-609.

Wilke WS (2001). Can fibromyalgia and chronic fatigue syndrome be cured by surgery? Cleveland Clinic Journal of Medicine, 68(4): 277-9.

Wolf DA, Veasey DA III, Wilson SK, Adame J, Korndorffer WE (1998). Death following minor head trauma in two adult individuals with the Chiari I deformity. Journal of Forensic Sciences. 43(6), 1241-1243.

Won DJ, Nambiar U, Muszynski CA, Epstein FJ (1997). Coagulation of herniated cerebellar tonsils for cerebrospinal fluid pathway restoration. Pediatric Neurosurgery, 27(5), 272-275.

Wynn R, Goldsmith, AJ (2004). Chiari type I malformation and upper airway obstruction in adolescents. <u>International Journal of Pediatric Otorhinolaryngology</u>. 68(5): 607-11.

Glossary of commonly used terms

Apnea- to stop breathing, often due to compression on the brainstem or lower cranial nerves.

Arachnoid- one of the membranes surrounding the brain and spinal cord. It appears to resemble a spider web. (There are 3 layers of covering of the brain and spinal cord- the dura, arachnoid and pia.)

Arachnoiditis- inflammation of the arachnoid membrane.

Aspirate- to inhale fluids, food products, or other materials into the lungs. Most often due to problems swallowing.

Asymptomatic- without symptoms. Someone who has no symptoms that can be attributed to a disorder.

Ataxia- inability to coordinate movement. Stumbling when walking, or inability to maintain a fluid gait when asked to walk a straight line.

Atrophy- wasting away of the muscle. Can be due to problems with the nerves going to the muscles.

Atrophic- changes in the muscle that create an appearance of being wasted away.

Basilar invagination- the base of the skull and the first cervical vertebra dent inward, causing pressure on the brainstem or upper cervical spinal cord.

Catheter- a small soft plastic tube used to drain fluid. For example, a Foley catheter is often inserted into the bladder to drain urine or a shunt catheter may be inserted into ventricles of the brain to drain spinal fluid and treat hydrocephalus.

Cerebellum- the lower part of the brain that lies in the posterior fossa and is responsible for coordination and fluidity of movement.

Cerebrospinal fluid- (CSF)- clear, water-like fluid that flows around the brain and spinal cord, and acts to bathe the structures. The total CSF volume in an adult is about 150ml (or about 1 pint).

Cervical- pertaining to the neck.

CINE MRI—a special MRI scan that looks at the flow of cerebrospinal fluid around the posterior fossa and into the spinal canal.

Chiari I Malformation—herniation of the cerebellar tonsils, and in some cases the lower part of the brainstem, into the upper cervical canal.

Clonus- abnormal, uncontrolled jerking of the foot when the ankle is flexed upward.

Cranial nerves- a set of 12 nerves in the brain that control motor and sensory functions.

Diplopia- symptom of seeing double, or double vision.

Dura mater- the tough outer covering surrounding the brain and spinal cord. Is located just inside the skull and the spinal canal.

Disequilibrium- inability to maintain proper balance. Often noted as stumbling or falling to one side.

Dysesthesia- an unpleasant sensation. A symptom of pins and needles or tingling when skin is touched.

Dysphagia- inability to swallow properly. Often leads to aspiration.

Ectopia- mild herniation, displacement or hang down of tissue.

Electrocautery- a small instrument that uses heat and is used in many surgeries to stop bleeding. May be used in severe cases of the Chiari malformation to shrink the tips of the cerebellar tonsils.

Hemisphere- When referring to the brain: one half of the upper brain or of the cerebellum.

Herniation- abnormal protrusion (or overhang) of tissue. Some MRI reports will read "herniation of the tonsils"- this means the tonsils are hanging down too far.

Hoffman's sign (or reflex)- an abnormal reflex that is tested by placing the fingers in a neutral position, and (painlessly) flicking the nail of the middle finger. If positive, the other fingers will abnormally flex in response.

Hydrocephalus- Abnormal, over filling of the CSF fluid pockets (ventricles) in the brain. Can cause symptoms such as headache, balance problems, incontinence and memory problems.

Hydrosyringomyelia- a fluid cavity in the spinal cord. May also be referred to as syrinx, or syringomyelia.

Incidental finding- a finding that is unexpected, or unrelated to symptoms. May refer to a person who has a finding on MRI, but has no symptoms.

Institutional Review Board (IRB)- a group of professionals who review research proposals and ensure that no harm will come to individuals who participate in research. All research must be approved by the IRB of the participating institution.

Laminectomy- removal of the roof bone (or posterior arch) of a vertebra.

Limb ataxia- inability to maintain fluid movement of the arm or leg. Inability to touch finger to nose properly.

Lumbar- referring to the lower most part of the spine.

Meninges- the 3 layers of covering that surround the brain and spinal cord. Consists of the dura mater, the pia mater and the arachnoid.

Meningitis- inflammation of the meninges. May be due to bacterial or viral infection.

Myelogram- special radiology study that involves injecting contrast material (like a dye) into the spinal canal and taking x-rays of where the contrast travels. The test is often followed by a CAT scan of the area and is done to determine if there is blockage of spinal fluid flow or if there is nerve or spinal cord compression. This test is less commonly used than MRI.

Myelomeningocele- herniation or protrusion of the spinal cord through a defect in development of the neural tube- seen in infants. Usually associated with Chiari type II.

Nystagmus- abnormal bobbing of the eyes that can be demonstrated when the person looks to the side or up and down.

Parasthesia- abnormal sensation in the extremity.

Pericranium- a tissue layer between the scalp and skull.

Periosteum- a tissue layer lining the bones of the body. In the skull, it is called pericranium.

Posterior fossa- A general term for the back area of the brain. This is where the brain stem, cerebellum, and cerebellar tonsils lie.

Shunt- small, soft plastic tube that is used to drain fluid.

Sleep apnea- to stop breathing intermittently when sleeping. Symptom can be described as waking up short of breath or gasping for air.

Syncope- Spells of passing out, or fainting (loss of consciousness). Different from a seizure.

Syringomyelia- abnormal fluid cavity in the spinal cord.

Syrinx- abnormal fluid cavity in the spinal cord.

Tethered cord- When the spinal cord becomes stuck to the surrounding structures or held under tension by the tough band at the bottom of the spinal cord called the filum terminale.

Thoracic- refers to the chest area. The thoracic spine is the part of the spine running from the top of the shoulders down to the beginning of the lower back.

Tinnitus- ringing in the ears.

Tonsillar ectopia- abnormal protrusion or hang down of the tonsil tissue of the cerebellum.

Tonsils- a small, often rounded mass of tissue. There are several types of tonsils in the body, including in the throat, in the intestine, and in the brain. In reference to the brain, indicates the tissue at the bottom of cerebellum.

Ventricle- fluid pocket within the brain where spinal fluid is created. There are four ventricles in the brain. Enlargement of the ventricles is called hydrocephalus.

INTERNET RESOURCES

The American Headache Society
www.americanheadachesociety.org

American Pain Foundation
www.painfoundation.org

The American Syringomyelia Alliance Project
www.asap.org

The Chiari Care Center
www.chiaricare.com

Chiari Connection International
www.chiariconnectioninternational.com

The Chiari Institute
www.chiariinstitute.com

Chiari People of Montana
www.chiaripeople.org

The Chiari Times
www.chiaritimes.com

Conquer Chiari
www.conquerchiari.org

e-Medicine: Chiari I Malformation
www.emedicine.com/radio/topic149.htm

e-Medicine: Chiari II Malformation
www.emedicine.com/radio/topic150.htm

The March of Dimes Birth Defects Foundation
www.marchofdimes.com/

The National Headache Foundation
www.headaches.org

The National Organization for Rare Disorders
www.rarediseases.org

The NINDS Chiari Malformation Information Page
www.ninds.nih.gov/disorders/chiari/chiari.htm

Spina Bifida Association of America
www.sbaa.org

The World Arnold Chiari Malformation Association
www.pressenter.com/-wacma/

Made in the USA
Columbia, SC
08 August 2021